I would encourage anyone to become one of the thousands whose lives have already been transformed by First Place. These profoundly simple but critical God-centered principles will bring a much-needed balance to your spiritual, mental, physical, and emotional health.

>Dr. James T. Draper, Jr.
>President, Baptist Sunday School Board

Carole Lewis' tireless efforts through the First Place program have led to the improved health and well-being of thousands. The First Place program has become a recognized resource for individuals and churches around the country. Now, *First Place* puts the principles of this effective program within the reach of multitudes more. It is destined to impact the vitality of the Church of Jesus Christ and the pursuit of her mission.

>Jim Florence, DrPH, CHES
>Assistant Professor, Dept. of Public Health
>East Tennessee State University, Johnson City, TN

Carole Lewis' love, passion, and commitment to First Place is a blessing to all of us whose lives have been touched by hers. More importantly, her zeal and availability have allowed the Lord to take a *dynamic program* and transform it into a Christ honoring *ministry* for so many. It always amazes me to see God use the improbable to do the seemingly impossible with each victory achieved, thanks to Carole and First Place.

>John Bernard
>Minister of Family Life
>First Baptist Church, Dallas, TX

Many changes have taken place in my life since I began facilitating First Place groups about six years ago. The physical and spiritual advantages of the program have made such a difference in my life and it is my privilege to share this with many others. I am grateful to God for making possible for me a "divine" appointment with Carole Lewis. That day began a pilgrimage for me in every area of my life. Discipline is no longer a negative word and accountability has become very important to me. I thank God for the First Place program and how it has taught me more about how to focus on God's will and how to rely on his infinite power in every circumstance.

>Irene Bonner
>Director, Cecil B. Day Wellness Center
>Dunwoody Baptist Church, Atlanta, GA

First Place is the finest program available for individuals concerned about being totally healthy. Other programs may produce faster (and short term) weight loss, but none leads to wholeness like First Place. It's health for the soul, mind, body, and spirit—it's the real thing!

>Dr. Bill Heston
>Vice President for University Advancement
>Howard Payne University

The First Place ministry has changed my life personally. It helps us put our faith in the places where we live and have our most difficult struggles. God has used the First Place program to produce some of the most committed Christians all across America. I have found entire churches in many states that have been transformed by First Place. I know of no other program that ministers to the whole person as thoroughly as the First Place program.

>Dr. Bobby Boyles
>Senior Pastor, Eagle Heights Church
>Oklahoma City, OK

I am so excited about this new book! And I'm excited about First Place! It is the healthiest way to lose weight *and* keep the spiritual atmosphere in our lives. Prayer *does* change things in our body, mind, and spirit!

>Marge Caldwell
>Author, Speaker, Marriage Counselor

As a member, I was able to lose (and maintain) 50 stubborn pounds. As a leader, I have seen God work intimately in the lives of men and women. *First Place* truly is life changing.

>Debbie DeaBueno
>Virtue Magazine

I joined First Place over three years ago because of a desire to lose weight. I am a chef and around food all day long, so you can imagine the trouble I can get into. As a certified professional chef, I am required to have thirty hours of training in both nutrition and sanitation. However, I learned more about nutrition and healthy eating in my first session of First Place than I did in my culinary classes. But, after only a couple of weeks the diet portion (or the "live-it" as we call it) became secondary to the spiritual food and blessings I was fed. I haven't reached my goal yet, but with the ingredients that I have been given, and with the Lord's help, I know that I have the right recipe for success.

>Scott Wilson, C.E.C., A.A.C.
>Chef/Owner, Healthy Home Cooking!

God has allowed me the wonderful privilege of watching thousands of people learn to walk with Him daily through First Place. I've enjoyed a relationship with the people in this life-changing program since its earliest stages and witnessed the kind of growth which can only be explained by God's approval and blessing. I joyfully testify to the biblical integrity of First Place and the spiritual authenticity of those in leadership. Carole Lewis is both a dear friend and an accountability partner to me. I have known her far too long not to know the real Carole! She is genuine, approachable, and absolutely convinced that God is not just the answer to our spiritual needs, but our emotional, mental, and physical as well. God's way works, beloved! It has worked for Carole, it has worked for me, and it will work for you!

>Beth Moore
>Author, Bible Study Teacher

First Place

First Place

The Original Spiritually Based
Weight-Loss Plan for Whole-Person Fitness

Carole Lewis
with W. Terry Whalin

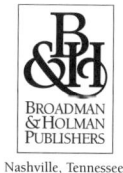

Broadman
& Holman
Publishers

Nashville, Tennessee

©1998
by Carole Lewis
All rights reserved
Printed in the United States of America

0-8054-0179-2

Published by Broadman & Holman Publishers, Nashville, Tennessee
Page Design: Desktop Miracles, Inc., Dallas, Texas
Editor: Janis Whipple

Dewey Decimal Classification: 613.2
Subject Heading: WEIGHT LOSS—RELIGIOUS ASPECTS—CHRISTIANITY. /
HEALTH—RELIGIOUS ASPECTS—CHRISTIANITY.
Library of Congress Card Catalog Number: 98-45914

Unless otherwise stated all Scripture citation is from the Holy Bible, New International Version, copyright © 1973, 1978, 1984 by International Bible Society. Other versions cited are: KJV, the King James Version; LB, The Living Bible, copyright © Tyndale House Publishers, Wheaton, Ill., 1971, used by permission; and the New Living Translation, copyright © 1996 Tyndale House Publishers, Wheaton, Ill., used by permission, all rights reserved.

Library of Congress Cataloging-in-Publication Data

Lewis, Carole, 1942–
    First place / Carole Lewis with W. Terry Whalin
      p. cm.
    ISBN 0-8054-0179-2 (pbk.)
    1. Weight loss—Religious aspects—Christianity. 2. Health—Religious aspects—Christianity. I. Whalin, Terry. II. Title.
RM222.2.L446   1997
613.2'5—dc21

98-45914
CIP

2 3 4 5 02 01 00 99 98

TABLE OF CONTENTS

ACKNOWLEDGMENTS
xi

INTRODUCTION
1

CHAPTER ONE
A Challenge for America
5

CHAPTER TWO
Putting God in First Place
15

CHAPTER THREE
Dig Down Deep—What's Your Motivation?
27

CHAPTER FOUR
Obstacles to Overcome
37

CHAPTER FIVE
The Spiritual Foundation
49

FIRST PLACE

CHAPTER SIX
Discovering Balance
61

CHAPTER SEVEN
The First Five Commitments
79

CHAPTER EIGHT
The Final Four Commitments
99

CHAPTER NINE
Beyond the Basics
129

CHAPTER TEN
A Dream for Tomorrow
135

APPENDIX A
Personal Testimonies
145

APPENDIX B
Live-It Food Exchanges
173

APPENDIX C
Fact Sheet Information
193

APPENDIX D
Breakfast—Why or Why Not?
201

APPENDIX E
Eating Out
205

Table of Contents

APPENDIX F
Recipes
207

APPENDIX G
Exercise Basics and Exercise Log
235

APPENDIX H
Sample Bible Study
261

APPENDIX I
First Place Resources
264

ENDNOTES
265

ACKNOWLEDGMENTS

Special thanks to our First Place staff in Houston. Your prayers and loving support give me the blessed opportunity to see what can happen in the workplace when Jesus is given First Place. Each of you are a shining example of what a Christian man and woman should be. I love you and it is my great joy to serve God with you.

To all the First Place members and leaders who love and pray for this ministry on a daily basis. Your changed lives are the tangible evidence that Christ truly has been given His rightful position . . . first place.

INTRODUCTION

What direction have you chosen for your life? Take a look beyond this day or this hour and look at the overall picture of your health—emotionally, physically, spiritually, and mentally. How do you measure up to your own expectations? More importantly, how do you evaluate yourself compared to God's standard? These complex questions have no simple answers.

Many years ago as a young married woman with three small children, I heard Dr. Ralph Neighbor, a missionary, discuss telling others about Jesus Christ. He said, "Witnessing is nothing but one hungry beggar telling another where to find the bread." Throughout the past twenty-five years, those words have been driven into my mind and heart, yet their meaning goes beyond how I share my faith with other people. For me, the Christian life symbolizes one hungry beggar telling another where to find the Bread—the Lord Jesus Christ. Jesus Himself said in John 6:35, "I am the bread of life. He who comes to me will never go hungry, and he who believes in me will never be thirsty." True satisfaction in life is only discovered as we hunger and thirst after Jesus Christ.

As we look for ways to overcome the obstacles we face we often search for the easy answers. Is it fast? Will I be able to do it quickly? What is the most efficient method? Words like *quick, time-saving, fast,*

FIRST PLACE

and *efficient* are advertising buzz words that power almost every consumer marketing effort. In our rapid-paced world, we select the quicker method or the faster way or the time-saving option. In 1945, Percy Le Baron Spencer invented the microwave oven. Today the microwave oven has transformed the way that many people prepare food. At the grocery store, we scan the back of a package to see if the product includes instructions for the microwave. If those instructions are on the package, we toss it into our shopping cart. If not, we slip it back on the shelf. Everyone is looking for a quick meal.

Our search for the quick and easy solution isn't confined to food. We look for the ten-minute devotion, the short-cut to work, and the fastest processor inside our computer. Because of my work, I have a cell phone, a pager, an e-mail address, as well as other gadgets. While this equipment increases my availability to my staff, it does not bring me fulfillment or satisfaction. True satisfaction can only be found in a daily relationship with the eternal God who is our refuge. Each day, I turn my life over to Christ and ask Him to speak through me and use my life as an example of Jesus for others. It's not easy, and it's fraught with mistakes. I am merely one hungry beggar writing the words in these pages. If you are looking for the quick and easy way, this isn't the book for you.

You will find that First Place is about a process where we fellow pilgrims are on a journey, learning more about how to follow Jesus every day. Our foundational Bible verse for the First Place program is Matthew 6:33. As He taught on the mountainside, Jesus Christ gave His most famous sermon called The Sermon on the Mount. As Jesus spoke to this weary crowd about the subject of worry and concern about God's guidance, He told them not to worry or be concerned. Jesus illustrates this by saying, "Look at the birds of the air; they do not sow or reap or store away in barns, and yet your heavenly Father feeds them. Are you not much more valuable than they?" But then He gave them (and us) the key for living out this life change, saying, "But seek first his kingdom and his righteousness, and all of these things will be given to you as well." Yet we, in our impatience, want the "things" without going through the first steps.

Introduction

You've selected this book for a reason. The "thing" you want may be to lose a specific amount of weight. Or possibly your goal with weight loss is to raise your self-esteem. Or maybe it's as practical as fitting into a swimsuit for the beach next summer. However, the critical question this book will address over and over is: Are you willing to go through the process of spiritual growth necessary to have these "things" added to your life?

The process involves turning to God every day, giving Him the highest priority—first place—in your every action. This act of setting God as a priority relates to more than good choice; it encompasses every decision and conversation throughout the day. Each of us needs to seek God's direction and guidance for our lives. After you've committed the situation to God, are you seeking His righteousness? The pages that follow contain some specific guidance about how to move along the path of seeking God's kingdom in all aspects of your life. Jesus wants to have first place.

Dear friend, as you read about the program we call First Place, I pray that it reveals more than simply another diet plan. When it comes to shedding pounds, most of us have already read enough information to lose every pound to get to our ideal weight. Instead, I pray you will discover my Friend, Jesus Christ. He is the Bread of Life. May God bless your search for the true Bread who can change your life—body and soul.

Carole Lewis
First Place National Director

Caution: Before undertaking this or any other weight loss program, you should consult your physician and disclose any pre-existing medical history which might effect your participation in the program including, but not limited to, heart disease, high blood pressure, anorexia/ bulimia, diabetes, or hypoglycemia.

CHAPTER ONE

A Challenge for America

Susan Crawford battled her weight since she was a child. Her weight problem escalated during her first pregnancy. After her baby was born, she remained 65 pounds overweight. Hurting and anxious about her weight, Susan began to face dealing with a troubled marriage as well. Her husband pleaded with her to lose the weight. She tried for twelve years through a variety of weight loss plans and lost weight, only to gain it again. Nothing seemed to help, and Susan's weight climbed to 257 pounds.

But something happened to Susan to help her face the root of her problem with food. On May 18, 1980, Susan received the news that her grandmother, whom she dearly loved, had died. Returning to work after a leave of absence, Susan sat in her car during lunchtime and attacked a bag of chocolate-covered wafer cookies as she privately continued to mourn her loss. As Susan reached for another cookie, suddenly she realized she was using food to deal with the grief of her loss. Susan now saw how she had been using food as a way of coping with her emotional needs. Only being a Christian for two years, Susan began to pray for a more permanent solution to her problems with food.

FIRST PLACE

That answer came a few months later when Susan read about a weight loss program that included Bible study in her church's newsletter. She joined the class and for the first time in her life felt the hope she needed to face her weight-loss challenge. Through First Place, a Christ-Centered Health Program, Susan had learned how to deal with the source of her unhealthy eating behaviors.

Did her marriage problems disappear as the pounds came off? Susan's weight was only one symptom of deeper marital issues. After Susan lost 60 of the 100 pounds she would eventually lose, she and her husband separated and later divorced. Susan says that her husband's decision to divorce made her question why she should continue to lose weight, but God gave her the strength to continue. She began to focus on her motivation for losing the weight. She learned that her desire to lose weight should come from wanting to please God and not to please her husband or herself.

Since Susan had experienced healing through First Place in early 1981, she was able to become a leader. For Susan to lead such a class was like one hungry beggar leading another to bread. She had a weight goal of 165 pounds, but unlike other weight loss organizations, Susan did not need to be at her goal before she could lead a group. Her only requirement was availability.

Today, Susan has been remarried for sixteen years and is the local First Place representative for Houston's First Baptist Church. She assists about thirty-five group leaders and the over 250 participants in these various groups come from a wide range of churches and denominations. In 1997, Susan wrote the First Place Bible study "Pathway to Success" that chronicles her journey to success. As you can see Susan achieved weight loss and more.

Dr. Dick Couey, physiologist at Baylor University, says, "Unless you keep the weight off for five years, you can't con-

A Challenge for America

sider the loss permanent." Susan learned that First Place involved more than weight loss—it was a total lifestyle change. Susan says, "Most of us want God to change us instantly. Instead, God wants to be magnified in our weaknesses and prove the sufficiency of His grace in our lives." She admits a daily dependence on God, saying, "He uses my weaknesses for His purposes."

In the following pages, you will learn how Susan and thousands of others have found a life change. No one suggests that such change will be simple or without cost—but the changes are possible if we are to become balanced people of God.

ENDLESS CHOICES RELATED TO FOOD

As a nation, America is full of fabulous grocery stores. The shelves are loaded with such variety that our minds spin when even trying to determine which type of cereal to buy. We have the largest selection of fresh vegetables, fruits, and meats in the world. For bread, we can choose fresh baked or processed breads from local bakeries. When it comes to dairy products, there are a variety of brands of milk, cheese, and yogurt. Canned goods and packaged items are in abundance, and the aisles of frozen foods seem endless.

Last summer, I talked with a young woman from Russia who attended one of our Fitness Weeks. I asked, "How did you feel the first time you went into a grocery store in our country?" To my surprise, she described how difficult it was selecting products here because she didn't have many choices available in her country. I thought the opportunity to select from such variety would have brought this Russian woman great joy, not confusion. Then it hit me—as Americans we are blessed with a variety of food; however, we are also confused by the endless choices.

FIRST PLACE

We received a letter from a missionary in Africa who is on the First Place program. It's a challenge for this missionary to make choices because of the lack of sugar-free items available. Her mother sends sugar-free items from America, but locally there are only two fresh fruit choices—pineapples and bananas. For her milk, this missionary has to purchase it from a local farm, and even after skimming it twice, it's still probably only one percent and not skim milk. Once again I was reminded of our abundance in America and our variety of food choices.

Besides our grocery stores, we have a restaurant on every corner. Even the smallest of towns has a couple of fast food restaurants and a local cafe. The variety of restaurants is endless. Americans can choose foods from anywhere in the world. We can take out or eat inside. Most of us have easy access to every kind of food imaginable.

America also has the finest medical facilities in the world. There are medical centers in every major city, with doctors who specialize in every illness known to man. Yet despite all these potential advantages, we still have the reputation of being the unhealthiest developed nation in the world. The five greatest health problems today are cancer, diabetes, heart disease, hypertension (high blood pressure), and lower back pain—and America leads the world in all of them. Health professionals tell us it is due to our poor eating habits and our sedentary lifestyles.

John Graham, director of Harvard's Center for Risk Analysis in Boston, says that "by changing personal behavior, people could reduce their risk of dying early by 70% to 80%." Professor Graham also says, "The number one and number three killers in America are heart disease and stroke, which often are caused by a fatty diet, failure to exercise, high cholesterol and high blood pressure. The number two and number four killers are cancer and lung disease, which may be brought on by the choices we make."[1]

Obesity increases the risk of diabetes, heart disease, high blood pressure, gallbladder disease, arthritis, breathing problems, and some forms of cancer. Poor diet and inactivity causes 300,000 deaths a year, according to a study published in the *Journal of the American Medical Association.*

A Challenge for America

Most Americans who are aware of their own obesity generally try dieting at one point or another. Many try losing the weight by going on crash diets found in their favorite magazines or books from their local bookstores. Others may try liquid diet plans where they deprive themselves of solid food and many times, the necessary nutrients for their bodies. However, studies of weight loss show that these type of crash diets in general don't work. As soon as a person ends a particular diet, the weight returns. Studies show that 95 percent of people who lose weight gain it back within two years.

A NATIONAL FIXATION ON WEIGHT LOSS

Every year, Americans spend $33 billion on weight-reduction programs and products, but they don't seem to do much good. The number of overweight Americans increased from 25 percent in 1980 to 33 percent in 1991. According to the National Health and Nutrition Examination Survey, 11 percent of children and adolescents are overweight, up from about 5 percent in the 1970s. At any given time, 33 to 40 percent of women are trying to lose weight and 20 to 24 percent of men are dieting.[2]

The weight loss craze is the second most popular recreational means of spending money, topped only by fitness. During the months of January and September, full-page newspaper ads lure us into one program or another to lose weight. Weight loss professionals understand that most Americans think about weight loss more during these two times of the year. New Year's resolutions spark the interest in January; people see this month of beginnings as a great time to lose any weight gained since Halloween. September is the second choice to lose weight before we stuff ourselves during the Thanksgiving and Christmas seasons.

As a society, we are now consumed with thoughts about weight and exercise. Many of us are on a search for a quick fix. At the same time, we are unwilling to consider permanent changes in our lifestyles.

FIRST PLACE

Some programs tell us to eat foods high in protein and low in carbohydrates to lose weight. Others advise the exact opposite. There are programs that tell us to eliminate certain food groups like milk and meat from our diet, while others say that the key to weight loss is to juice our fruits and vegetables and eat everything raw for optimum health. Another program teaches that God created every food, and if we pray and study our Bible but still want Ding Dongs or Twinkies, that's OK; we just need to stop eating when full. Other programs sell us our food; our only task to lose weight is to heat and eat those foods. The problem with this method is that we still have to learn to prepare nutritious food after we have lost the weight.

Some men and women have taken drastic measures to lose weight—such as having a physician staple their stomach. Then they can only consume a couple of tablespoons of food at one time. However, even with these severe measures, many people still find ways to eat enough and remain overweight. Another alarming weight loss method is the use of drugs to curb the appetite. In the 1960s and 1970s, diet pills were prescribed to those wanting to lose weight; they were amphetamines. Amphetamines suppressed appetite; however, they made those who took them wired and addicted. Other drugs replaced amphetamines. These new drugs increased brain chemicals that affected moods and suppressed the appetite.

The sales for diet pills took off again in 1992 when University of Rochester researchers reported the results of a three-and-a-half-year study of patients using a combination of fenfluramine and phentermine (fen-phen). Patients lost weight for six months and then saw their weight level off. At the end of the study, patients had lost an average of fifteen pounds from their starting weight. In 1996, doctors in the United States issued 18 million prescriptions for fen-phen. In 1997, the Mayo Clinic and the Food and Drug Administration announced that the combination of these two drugs may deform heart valves and cause irreversible lung damage. In late 1997, the FDA recalled the diet drugs Redux and fenfluramine—one half of the fen-phen drug cocktail. Many of the six million patients who used them had to quit cold turkey.

A Challenge for America

Almost every day in the newspaper and news magazines, so-called authorities bombard us with health information, telling us that if we don't do it their way, then we are doomed to failure or a lifetime of poor health. Since pesticides are killing us, we are cautioned to buy only organic meats and produce. Other news articles proclaim that our foods have no vitamins left so we must megadose on vitamin and mineral supplements. We are left not sure what is factual and what is not.

This plethora of weight loss programs and information stirs mass confusion about how to take weight off and lose it permanently. We then look in the mirror and see we are still fat despite losing hundreds of pounds in our lifetime.

What can be done?

WHAT IS A SAFE WEIGHT LOSS PROGRAM?

To help us sort through the confusion surrounding weight loss, we turned to Dick Couey, a professor of health sciences at Baylor University and a physiologist who has studied nutrition and how it relates to the biochemistry of the cell. On a regular basis, Dr. Couey gives his opinion about the safety or effectiveness of certain diets. His criteria for a good diet includes:

1. The diet must contain the forty-five known nutrients in their proper amounts. It must contain enough carbohydrate, fat, protein (especially nitrogen), nine amino acids, thirteen vitamins, nineteen minerals, and sufficient amounts of water.
2. The diet should contain at least 1,200 calories per day. Caloric consumption below 1,200 could possibly cause damage to your body and permanently lower its basal metabolism.
3. The diet should emphasize behavior modification techniques to overcome poor eating habits or problem eating. It should also stress ways to make lifestyle changes in order to facilitate weight maintenance and thwart further weight gain.

4. The diet should not only stress good eating practices, but also emphasize regular physical activity, stress reduction, and other healthy changes in lifestyle. In addition, Dr. Couey recommends a Christian emphasis to help motivate participants to properly care for his or her body.

"Be very careful about choosing other nutritional programs. Many of these programs are designed to help you lose weight; however, they may lack the proper amounts of nutrients which can damage the health of the cell," concludes Dr. Couey.

After listing these four criteria, Dr. Couey includes a final caution about selecting a diet program. "Fad diets usually don't work because they are not designed for permanent weight loss. Habits are not changed, and the food selection is so limited that the person cannot follow the diet for more than two or three weeks. Although dieters assume they have lost fat, they have actually lost mostly muscle and other lean tissue mass. In a matter of weeks, most of the lost weight is back. The dieter appears to have failed, when actually the diet failed. The whole scenario can add more blame and guilt to the psyche of the dieter, which is very unfortunate."

In his final bit of advice, Dr. Couey extends hope, saying, "If someone needs help losing weight, First Place is the answer. My wish for you is expressed beautifully in 3 John 2 which says, 'I pray that you may enjoy good health and that all may go well with you, even as your soul is getting along well.'"

HOPE AHEAD

When it comes to weight loss, you may wonder if anyone can find hope. Yes, I believe you can. In the chapters that follow, I will detail a program called First Place. After an initial overview of the program along with my personal experience and several others, we will look at motivation and the various obstacles to weight loss. Next we will consider what the Bible has to do with a weight loss program and why it is

A Challenge for America

critical to have a spiritual foundation to a weight loss program. First Place is more than weight loss—it's a lifestyle change that encourages every participant to find balance in his or her own life. Balance is the topic for a separate chapter. The third and final section of the book examines the First Place program in detail. This section includes some ready-to-use tools and nine distinct commitments that are a part of the program. I'll also detail additional possibilities beyond the basic program, such as fitness weeks, conferences, and training programs. In the final pages of this book, we will look beyond weight loss specifics—I want to give you a great dosage of hope and a plan for lifestyle changes that show you the reality of Jesus in everyday life.

While the text portion of this book finishes in an uplifting fashion, it's not the final page of the book. Don't ignore the appendixes at the back of the book. They are loaded with helpful information such as recipes; stories of people from First Place, including their before and after photos; the food exchange list; and a variety of resources to help you begin a First Place group.

Throughout my years with First Place, I've met numerous people who have lost more than a hundred pounds using this program. Initially I am amazed at the transformation in a single individual; such a weight loss seems impossible. Then I remember that these people didn't lose their weight overnight; they did it over a period of months or years. What's more, they are keeping that weight off—permanently. You may be scared to take such a journey or even to entertain the possibility of losing weight permanently. If so, consider the Chinese proverb that says, "The journey of a thousand miles begins with a single step."

Turn the page and let's take the first step to learn about the First Place program.

CHAPTER TWO

Putting God in First Place

At age four, Karen Arnett spent a few months with her grandparents. When her parents arrived to take her home, they hardly recognized Karen because she had gained so much weight. As she says, "My grandmother fed me very well." Despite Karen's active childhood, she remained overweight.

Today when Karen considers the main reason she overate, she says it was from boredom. "If I was having a bad day with the kids or a financial problem or a fight with my husband, I ate," she says. Food was Karen's reward and comfort. Her weight steadily increased to 416 pounds. At her home in Evans, Georgia, Karen started a low-fat diet plan in December 1994 and lost 68 pounds. While the low-fat plan was helping, she knew it wasn't the total answer to her health needs. Karen says, "I wasn't submitting my life to God completely. I still overate and didn't exercise."

In May 1995, Karen started the First Place program and now sees how God has blessed every area of her life. Her dress size has gone from a 56 to a 10/12 and Karen has lost $83\frac{1}{2}$ inches and a total of 261 pounds. Since January 1997, Karen has maintained her weight at 155 pounds. A shy person by nature, at one time Karen found it difficult to say anything and usually stood in the back of a room. "It wasn't until I found First Place that I realized only God could truly help me. Only by committing all of my life to Him and disciplining myself could I overcome my eating problems," Karen says. Through the program her life has changed drastically, and Karen sees this change as evidence of God's power. "When I was overweight, I was not a testimony to God and His power in my life. Now God has used the weakest area of my life to exhibit His power."

WHAT IS FIRST PLACE?

Since the First Place program began in 1981, it has spread to all fifty states and over 12,000 churches from various denominations. First Place is also active in at least thirteen foreign countries. Yet most of you have probably never heard of First Place. It has no huge advertising budget or marketing efforts to get the word out about the program. Those of us involved in First Place have given the program over to God for His glory, and I often say God is our "publicist." Most of the growth has come from word-of-mouth and the enthusiasm of people who have been through the program.

It all began during the late 70s. A group of Christians in the First Baptist Church in Houston, Texas, had one question: "Since God has saved us from our sins and given us an abundant life, why can't we, as Christians, use that same power in the area of weight control?" These people recognized that the spiritual life involved discipline. It takes discipline to pray and follow God every day. By the same token, it takes discipline to control our food consumption. The key desire of these Christians was to create a Christ-centered weight control program. With this firm goal in mind, they faced it—fully unaware of the immensity of the assignment.

Putting God in First Place

The program would focus totally on Christ and include Bible study, small-group support, a proven common-sense nutrition plan, a method of record keeping and many other elements. These early leaders knew that the key was to keep Christ first in every aspect of the program. And weight loss was not their only focus; they aimed to grow in every area of life: spiritual, mental, emotional, and physical. A key concept of the program was—and is—balance. (This topic will be covered in greater detail in chapter 6.)

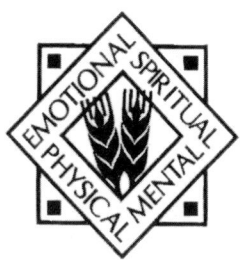

The logo for First Place illustrates the balance of the program. Each of the four aspects of life are given equal importance. The center of the logo has two shafts of wheat. It is representative of bread, which is significant throughout the Bible as God's provision. Jesus said in John 6:35, "I am the bread of life. He who comes to me will never go hungry." Through Christ, we can achieve balance in all four areas of life if we depend on Him daily to satisfy our "hunger." Jesus also taught that God's Word is central to achieving this by saying in Matthew 4:4, "It is written: 'Man does not live on bread alone, but on every word that comes from the mouth of God.'" Through studying God's Word we find that it provides guidelines for our physical well being, directs us spiritually, and equips us mentally to manage our busy lives. When we are students of His word, God also provides emotional stability by giving us understanding of His precepts and the ability to apply them in crisis and everyday situations through the Holy Spirit.

If you are facing physical hunger, as you pray to God, He can provide for your daily physical needs. If you are facing spiritual or emotional or mental hunger, the Bible is also the answer to your needs.

FIRST PLACE

The First Place program includes a series of nine commitments which will be explained in detail in chapters 7 and 8. In brief, these commitments include:

1. *Regular attendance in a small weekly meeting.* A key part of this program is commitment to a small group of people for a thirteen-week study. This group will be critical as you keep the other eight commitments; therefore, it is essential that you attend every meeting and stay for the entire session. (If you cannot locate a group or begin a group in your area, you will need to find 2 or 3 other friends to help you with accountability to the program.)

2. *Prayer.* As you pray every day at the same time, it will help you keep Christ first place in your life. God is concerned about your eating habits and food consumption. Prayer will be critical before you are tempted to eat the wrong food and prayer will see you through every day. As you communicate with God, you will build a closer relationship with your heavenly Father. Prayer is also an important part of the First Place meetings where group members pray for each other's needs every week.

3. *Bible reading.* The Bible says in John 8:32, "You will know the truth, and the truth will set you free." So often we avoid the truth from God's Word, yet this commitment is essential for spiritual growth. Regular reading from the Bible provides the foundation for a spiritual fitness plan. The First Place Scripture reading plan includes a daily Bible reading from the Old and New Testament. Each day's reading can be thoughtfully read in fifteen to thirty minutes.

4. *Scripture memory.* First Place involves memorizing a Bible verse each week and repeating it daily. The memory verse connects to the Bible lesson and provides daily strength and encouragement. God's Word in your heart will strengthen your daily life and spiritual relationship.

5. *Bible study.* This ten-week study is not meant to be intense. Every day you should read, meditate, and answer a small portion of that week's Bible study. Regular Bible study will build your spiritual fitness as you build your physical fitness.

6. *"Live-It."* The word *diet* sounds too morbid for a Christian program. When Christ is first place, the Christian life is meant to be lived abundantly. In First Place we use the word *Live-It* instead of *diet* (die-it). Through this commitment, you learn balanced eating habits. In Appendix B, I explain the size of a portion which we call an "exchange." The food exchange list is similar to one recommended by the American Diabetic Association and the foods are divided into six different groups: milk, vegetables, fruit, bread, meat, and fat. In First Place, we ask you to give up sugar until you reach your weight goal. Sugar includes honey and we'll explain the reason for this decision in Appendix B. Also we encourage you to reduce salt and caffeine. Following these food exchanges will be critical to your weight loss.

7. *Fact Sheet.* The Fact Sheet increases your awareness of what you eat each day. At first, the Fact Sheet may seem time-consuming, but actually it should only take a few minutes. The Fact Sheet builds accountability into the overall First Place program and helps you more easily control your calorie intake. Also the daily record reveals patterns of eating in a concrete fashion. Each week if you are attending a group, the Fact Sheet is turned in to your small group leader. Your leader then helps you with any problem you might be having by going to your Fact Sheet and evaluating your week of eating. You might also evaluate your Fact Sheets to detect any patterns you see.

8. *Phone call.* You make a commitment to call someone in your group every week. The phone call gives you a chance to call someone else in your group when you are tempted and ask them for prayer. Sometimes you may feel great and not need to call anyone; however, the name of someone will come into your mind. The Holy Spirit may be prompting you to call this person and encourage them. Many times, the person you call is feeling discouraged and even in the process of overeating.

9. *Exercise.* This commitment is based on 1 Corinthians 3:16 which says, "Don't you know that you yourselves are God's temple and God's Spirit lives in you?" What is the condition of God's house—your body? Are you ashamed of its size? If your body needs fixing, now is the time

to do it. You cannot expect to maintain any degree of physical fitness without some sort of exercise program. Aerobic exercise may mean joining an organized aerobic exercise class. Or you could walk briskly, jog, or bicycle several miles. Swimming is also an excellent aerobic exercise if you have joint problems. To get fit, you will need to exercise four or five times a week; to maintain fitness, you will need to exercise three times a week.

You may be saying to yourself, "Nine different commitments! Wow, how will I ever manage to keep all nine?" It may look overwhelming, but these key ingredients are necessary, if you desire to put Christ first place in your life. Most of us will not be able to do all nine commitments every day, but do strive to adhere to the commitments as much as you can, relying on the strength God provides. These commitments are our goal and when we reach this goal, it will bring balance into our lives. I heard it said once like this: "God loves us just the way we are, but too much to let us stay that way." An encouraging thought, isn't it?

When you do commit to God, expect the unexpected. Romans 8:29 says that God wants us to conform to the image of Jesus Christ. God wants to infiltrate every area of our life, and we believe that First Place covers every major area of life. As change occurs, it can be quite dramatic. Frequently I meet men and women who say they initially joined First Place to lose weight. Yet after they reached their weight goal, these same people say the most significant changes in their life were actually spiritual. As we put Jesus Christ in first place, many unexpected blessings will flow into our lives. With God's help we can grow every day to be more like Jesus Christ.

WHY AM I IN FIRST PLACE?

As the director of the First Place program since 1987, the passion of my life is to follow Jesus Christ every day. However, this passion wasn't there when I initially learned about First Place.

In 1980 I attended a baby shower and I saw my friend Kay for the first time in several years. Although we had grown up together and shared many experiences, I now saw that something had changed. I said, "Kay, how could you do this to me?"

She looked a bit puzzled and said, "Do what?"

I continued, "How could you lose weight and not tell me?"

Kay smiled and said, "Carole, have you forgotten that we are going to be forty next year? Do you want to be fat and forty?"

Her honesty shocked me. I had never combined the words *fat* and *forty*. For many years I had tried repeatedly to lose twenty pounds. When I was thirteen years old, I started dieting and from there I tried almost every available weight-loss plan. Over the years I seemed to gain and lose the same twenty pounds. I could not keep these twenty pounds from returning on any plan I tried. My conversation with Kay reminded me of this vicious cycle and I thought, *Here I am again, with the same twenty pounds and yes, I'm going to be forty next year.*

In Jeremiah 29:11 God said, "I know the plans I have for you" declares the LORD, "plans to prosper you and not to harm you, plans to give you hope and a future." Little did I know when I read in our church paper about a new weight-loss program called First Place that it would be there that God would begin His plans for my change. As I attended the First Place orientation, I thought to myself, *I am not all that sure that God cares much about my losing weight.* I thought He must be interested in much bigger things. However, I reminded myself of what Kay had said about being fat and forty and I registered for that first session.

I believe God did want me to lose those twenty pounds, but He also saw my inner rebellion. He would use First Place and the small group accountability there to help me surrender much more to Him. As I began the program, I didn't see the need to follow the food plan because I had lost weight with a low-carbohydrate diet previously. I thought to myself, *Why try something different?* I did not eat any bread or fruit, and I ate only four or five different kinds of vegetables with all the meat and fat I wanted, as long as it added up to 1,200 calories. At the meetings, my leader would evaluate my Fact Sheet with dismay, and write, "Carole, what are you doing?" In hindsight, I now see

FIRST PLACE

that not doing the food plan was another sign of my unwillingness to surrender to God's control.

I eventually ended up losing twenty pounds because I stayed within the 1,200 calories a day, despite my leader's encouragement to change my food habits. Although I was not eating by the program's Live-It food plan, I still loved the Bible study and fellowship and was content to stay with it. My success with losing the weight caught the attention of Dottie Brewer, one of the founders of the program. My First Place leader at that time then told Dottie that I had leadership potential. That is when I was asked to become a First Place leader myself. Petrified that I now had to teach a food plan that I did not know or follow, I began frantically to learn all I could to teach it. I did finally learn it and began teaching a Tuesday women's class in September 1981.

For three years, I led a class in my own strength. However, things began to change in my life. I was about to undergo a tremendous amount of turmoil. Because the Houston economy bottomed out during these years, our family was undergoing financial difficulties. My husband worked hard to save his business, but finally had to let go of it in 1984. In the process, we lost everything except our home. As an independent person, I had not had to depend on anyone. Suddenly I did not have a car so I had to depend on other people for my transportation.

I went to work in the education department at my church, First Baptist Houston in August 1984. Our family was at a low point in our lives. In mid-December of that year, God showed me that all our family had been going through was a means to draw me to Him—to give up my rebellious ways and let Him become Lord of everything about me.

Many years earlier, I had given my life to Jesus Christ and I called him Lord, but in reality, I had no idea how to let God be the Lord of my life. How could I give my life to God when I had been running it on my own for so many years? God was to answer my question a couple of weeks later when our pastor, Dr. John Bisagno, preached a sermon on the will. He said, "You might be here this morning and you know God wants to change your will. God will not come in and work

Putting God in First Place

on your will without your permission. If you will just pray this prayer this morning, 'Lord, I'm not willing but I'm willing to be made willing', then God will have permission to work on your will."

That Sunday morning, with the greatest sincerity I could muster, I prayed, "Lord, that's where I am today. I'm scared to death of what you might do with my life if I give you control of every part. But it can't be any worse than the way it is right now. My family is in a terrible mess and I feel like I'm such a mess spiritually and emotionally. So I give you permission to work on my will." Then I tacked a P.S. onto my prayer, "And please, God, don't let it hurt too much." In my mind, if someone was at the center of God's will, it had to be painful. For me, the most painful choice would be if God sent me to Africa or China since I certainly didn't want to go there. While I had no idea where God would take my simple prayer, I had found the key to change. I was willing to be willing. Many choices came later but this choice was the starting place.

In October 1984, I began a walking program; then three months later I started jogging. Today over thirteen years later, I continue jogging five times a week. This type of consistency was impossible—even in my dreams—when I started First Place. Throughout my entire life, I had never been consistent at anything! Everything I attempted was a start and stop proposition. God wanted to see consistency in many different areas where I failed to follow through. I love the patience and long-suffering of our Heavenly Father. Bit by bit, God gets the job done in our lives as we allow Him to work. Besides this area of exercise, God was teaching me to trust Him completely. It was a great lesson in my life about the importance of relationships.

A year before my personal crisis, the First Place program was beginning to move beyond First Baptist Houston. Some of the people who had completed the First Place program in our church had moved to other churches. They were asking, "How can we do First Place in our new church? This program is too wonderful to give up."

At the time, First Place didn't have a full-time staff person and Dottie Brewer, the founder of the program, was volunteering twenty to

FIRST PLACE

thirty hours a week. She was a person who jumped into a situation and got the job done. In the early years, First Baptist Houston had to loan us money to get started. Dottie made sure this money was returned and First Place was able to stand on its own.

In 1984, she presented the program to a Dallas publisher and proposed selling the program to them. They wanted to make it available to the public through the Christian bookstores. However, on the way back to Houston, Dottie was praying and felt God wanted to keep the program at First Baptist Houston. Dottie was concerned that people would use the book without one key ingredient, the small group accountability. (Though it is not necessary to be in a First Place small group for the rest of the program to work effectively, the importance of accountability is crucial for support. Therefore if a small group is not available in your area, the First Place program recommends you meet with two or three friends to keep accountable.) Dottie felt if someone bought a book about First Place in a bookstore, they would try the program without even seeking the support of a group. Instead, she felt it would be better if the program grew at a slower pace so she and the others could train leaders to use it properly. As people asked about First Place, we helped them start a program and by July 1987, the program had spread to about fifty churches.

The secretary who handled the clerical duties related to First Place was planning to take a maternity leave. The church's Minister of Activities approached me about taking over the First Place program. He was confident that I loved the program and would take over as the director of First Place. My initial months as the director of First Place were extremely hectic. I took orders for materials, opened the new accounts and shipped the materials, then followed through with billing. Over time, the church hired more staff to help me with the ordering and customer service. We created numerous resources and made them available. Then in 1992, Lifeway Press became our publisher. These resources, such as the First Place member notebook, Bible studies, video, the Leader's Guide, a cookbook, a prayer journal, an exercise log and others are listed in Appendix I.

Putting God in First Place

When I stepped into the position of director, I had no idea of the heartbreak that was ahead. In the fall of 1987, Dottie became ill and despite numerous tests, the doctors couldn't diagnosis her illness. In July 1988, they diagnosed colon cancer and Dottie lived another eight months. Along with Kay Smith, who later became my associate, I spent many hours at Dottie's bedside. Whenever Dottie wanted us at her bedside, we were there. Through her life, I learned about the consistency of Dottie's prayer life and the depth of her spirituality. God also worked in my heart during this time of pain and grief.

Dottie's body deteriorated; she had been an exercise walker for fifteen years and she could walk a fifteen-minute mile. When Dottie and I began exercising together, I had to jog beside her because of the fast walking pace. Now in the hospital, Dottie's heart was strong but her body was frail and weak. However, Dottie never lost her sense of humor. About three weeks before her death, propped up on some pillows and reflecting on how it all began, Dottie told me, "Carole, of all people, I would never have chosen you as the director of First Place." We had a good laugh about God's unusual sense of humor. I am sure she marveled at how God uses those who surrender late in life, or anytime, for His glory. She went home to be with the Lord on March 22, 1989. In many ways, First Place continues as a legacy to Dottie Brewer.

In my years as the director of First Place, the program has exploded in growth and includes the creation of many products to support our program. My starting point was certainly not very glorious, yet God was present in every decision. From the moment we accept Jesus as our personal Savior, God promises to invade our lives and never leave us. As we yield our lives into God's capable hands, He molds us into the person that we need to be. My daily passion with the First Place program has been to follow God's leading and will for my life. I'm willing to be willing.

What about your will? Are you willing to be willing? You've picked up this book and have read this far because you have a need in your life. God wants to fill that void in your total life picture—physically, emotionally, mentally, and spiritually.

FIRST PLACE

In the next chapter we want to examine motivations. What is the proper motivation for lifestyle choices and habits? What are improper motivations and how do we overcome them? Let's turn the page and take another step along our journey to wholeness in God's eyes.

CHAPTER THREE

Dig Down Deep— What's Your Motivation?

At the orientation session for First Place, Bill Patterson was worried. He felt like his life was a spiritual mess. As a Christian for almost nine years, Bill had never taken a single problem to the Lord. "While I was confident that I was a Christian, there was a huge spiritual gulf in my life," Bill says. "I never read the Bible and only prayed in public when I was forced to do so. We regularly attended church, but I had no active faith."

Weight loss was the major reason Bill joined a First Place group. "I didn't know how to eat, and when it came to convenience food, I was worse than everyone else, eating bags of chips and fried food," he says. "Food was essential for any celebration—a birthday, Christmas, or just getting together with friends." Bill had been heavy for most of his life, but he wasn't sure exactly how heavy until he joined a First Place group.

"It had been almost ten years since I had stepped on a scale," Bill admitted. "I knew my weight had increased and I thought it would be around 300, but I had no idea it would be 310 pounds the first night." Like many people, Bill wanted to deny there was a problem with his weight. One means to accomplish that denial was to avoid stepping on a scale. Every

FIRST PLACE

First Place meeting begins with the individuals weighing in. Members also may recite their memory verse for the week when they step on the scale.

Bill started the program in June 1996 along with his wife, Angie. Both of them have lost weight and are maintaining their weight goals. Bill went from 310 pounds to 185 pounds—he lost 125 pounds in ten months on the First Place program. An Exxon businessman, Bill travels from time to time. Because his driver's license photo now looks completely different, he gets a lot of questions at the airline counter, "What has happened to you?"

"I've had the opportunity to tell hundreds of people about what Christ has done in my life," Bill says. Before First Place, Bill lacked self-confidence in his work as well as in his witness for Christ. Since losing weight, and because of his active involvement in the Bible study, prayer, and other commitments of First Place, his spiritual life has been transformed. "God took control of my life, and now I know that I can take a step of faith in any situation," Bill says with a smile. "I'm quick to turn my problems over to the Lord, and I know that He will take care of them."

In 1996, Bill's parents noticed the change in him. They asked him how he and Angie had lost the weight. They shared with his parents the First Place program. Here's the interesting twist to this story. Bill's parents were not active in church. Not only did Bill and Angie lose wight, but Bill's parents returned to an active faith and now are regular church attenders.

WRONG REASONS FOR MAKING A LIFESTYLE CHANGE

Throughout this book, I describe a holistic program of lifestyle change for better health and weight loss. You're reading these pages for

Dig Down Deep—What's Your Motivation?

a reason, and it is important to examine *why* you want to make a lifestyle change. In this chapter, we're going to consider both wrong motivations and proper motivations. As part of the proper motivation, we will consider God's vision for why you should make a lifestyle change and look at three reasons to stay motivated.

The various wrong motivations are important to examine. As you consider these different reasons, pause every paragraph and see if that motivation is *your* motivation. If it is, then you are almost doomed to continue in your present state. These motivations have one unifying factor—they are temporary and are usually centered on another person.

Perhaps you are headed to a class reunion in a few months. Reunions are notorious for using photos of how we looked in high school on the name badges. How different do you look from that picture taken your senior year in high school? Most of us have changed substantially through the years. Our hairstyle is different as well as our overall physical appearance. You may set weight loss as a goal for this reunion and work toward it. The problem is the motivation is temporary.

Maybe one of your children is getting married in a few months, and you realize that you will be in the wedding pictures. Because of your social role in this situation, you will garner more attention and focus than you have in recent months. You stare down at your midsection and decide it's time to lose some pounds. Again, it's a temporary motivation.

Some husbands try to motivate their wives to lose weight by dangling a financial carrot. They sweetly look at their wives and say, "Honey if you lose fifty pounds then you can spend five hundred dollars on a new wardrobe." The thought of shopping for new outfits—in smaller sizes—is enticing, but let's look at the message underneath: "You are not OK. You don't look OK, and you would look a lot better if you didn't weigh so much. In fact, I'm backing that idea with my billfold and an investment in your clothes."

Another motivation may be the way others treat you. One of the worst things you can say to an overweight person is, "You have a pretty face." What sort of compliment is that? Although it may be the first thing that comes to mind, to an overweight person, such a comment is insulting. The real meaning behind those words translates, "If you would lose weight, you would be a knockout." If you want to compliment an overweight person, then focus on an internal character trait. Don't use their outward appearance as a motivator because the result will be temporary.

Many single people hope to lose weight because they think it will magically transform their social life. They mistakenly believe that a particular person will ask them for a date or that they will be able to ask a person out if they are slim. Unfortunately, this single individual is headed for disappointment because this is another improper motivation for shedding pounds.

If you are motivated to lose weight so you can please someone else—a spouse, a parent, a friend—then what happens when that relationship changes or has a barrier in it? You will return to eating like you have always eaten before.

A PROPER MOTIVATION

If you are extremely overweight, your goal may be to simply sit in a chair at the movies without bruising your thighs. Or you may want to travel on an airplane without asking a flight attendant for an extender for the seat belt.

You've tried to crack the whip and get those pounds off. It hasn't worked because every motivation that we've examined thus far has been temporary. Let's now look at what we at First Place consider to be proper motivations for successful, permanent weight loss.

Consider a Lifestyle Change

A key emphasis in First Place is a total lifestyle change. We're not looking for the quick solution, but a slow and steady process of change. Instead of attempting to lose thirty to forty pounds in a few weeks, First Place intentionally encourages a loss of one-and-a-half to two pounds per week. If you lose more than that amount, you are losing

Dig Down Deep—What's Your Motivation?

more than fat and are probably involved in a program that is not nutritionally sound. After the first few weeks of water loss, it is physiologically impossible to lose more than two pounds of fat per week.

Give Your Body to God

Get up and look in the mirror—you may not like what you see. A proper motivation is to give your body to God. You may think, *"God isn't interested in my body."* In Romans 12:1–2, the apostle Paul writes,

> "Therefore, I urge you, brothers, in view of God's mercy, to offer your bodies as living sacrifices, holy and pleasing to God—which is your spiritual worship. Do not conform any longer to the pattern of this world, but be transformed by the renewing of your mind. Then you will be able to test and approve what God's will is—his good, pleasing and perfect will."

We are urged to present our bodies to God as a living sacrifice. The people in the New Testament knew about sacrifice. Every day in the temple, animals were slaughtered and the blood was dripped on the altar as a sacrifice. As a part of our spiritual worship of God, we are called to present our bodies to God. Yes, the Lord cares about our physical bodies. A proper motivation for weight loss and total lifestyle change is to give your body to God. Ask for His transforming power to fill your life. It's a daily process and a key part of our motivation for pleasing God.

First Corinthians 6:19–20 says, "Do you not know that your body is the temple of the Holy Spirit, who is in you, whom you have received from God? You are not your own; you were bought at a price. Therefore honor God with your body." While it's sometimes easy to forget the fact, none the less it is true that we have the Spirit of God inside our bodies. As the temples in ancient Corinth housed false gods of stone and wood, Paul used the image of a temple to talk about how God's Spirit lives in our hearts. How are you taking care of your temple?

Sure, our problems in life have not disappeared. We still have financial struggles, problems in our workplace, and relational struggles; but our first priority and proper motivation is to turn to God and seek

His kingdom. As we put God in first place for our day and with our weight, then everything else falls into place.

Be a Role Model for Others

Many children are overweight and need encouragement from their parents. Another proper motivation for weight loss is to be a leader in your family and a role model for your children and spouse. It is impossible to lead people where you have not been yourself. The weight problems of our children would evaporate if we would lead them by example. My children and grandchildren love to walk or jog with me in the morning for exercise. Would they do it on their own? No way! Yet in a heart beat, they come with me at my invitation. If you can move away from the television set and walk together as a family, it will allow more time for conversation without the interruption of phones and other machines—plus you are working on one of the commitments in First Place—exercise.

Seek Emotional Healing

Weight loss may only be like an emotional band-aid. In some cases, you may come to First Place to lose weight when actually those extra pounds are only a symptom of a deeper issue. Women and men who have been emotionally or sexually abused often attempt to hide their pain with food and weight gain. We have several First Place groups that are specifically for the emotionally damaged. In these particular groups, members follow the First Place meeting schedule, then add an additional hour for deeper sharing. God is interested in every aspect of our lives—including our weight. Unless these people dig down to the deeper issues in their life, their weight loss is like putting a band-aid on cancer. It's not enough.

Stress Management

We live in a high-stress society. Almost every time we turn around, someone asks us to do something else. Our responsibilities pile high at the office, at home, and at church. A proper motivation for weight loss

Dig Down Deep—What's Your Motivation?

is to better manage the stress in life. It's clear to me that as we get our weight, nutrition, and exercise under control, our stress level becomes more tolerable. Although I have a stressful job, with twenty-five employees and a heavy travel schedule, I do not suffer from stress. I believe there are four reasons for this:

1. I have a daily quiet time with God each morning where I give the day to Him. He is in charge of my time and schedule.
2. I exercise five days a week. While running, I solve problems and plan my day.
3. I am not a worrier. As a child I learned from my mother that the things we worry about never happen. I believe worry is a great stress producer.
4. I get plenty of rest and take time off to play. Rest and leisure time are prerequisites to a stress-free life.

THREE WAYS TO KEEP MOTIVATED

As you start the journey of First Place, it is important to maintain motivation. One of the most common questions our leaders are asked is, "How do you stay motivated?" Here are three steps for staying motivated that have helped me.

1. *Act the way you want to feel.* Zig Ziglar, in his book *See You at the Top*, wrote that it's easier to act your way into a new way of feeling than it is to feel your way into a new way of acting.[1] We need to focus our minds on moving ahead—even when we don't feel like it. I find that this focus will change my feelings about a particular task. For example, some days I don't feel like exercising. A thousand and one excuses crowd into my mind, and if I went with my feelings, I'd just skip it. However, instead of giving in and skipping, I change into my exercise clothing and get out on the track. My feelings follow my actions. The same is true for any regular discipline, such as having my quiet time each day with the Lord or choosing to eat right: if I take action, then

my feelings follow. As you take continuous action for at least thirty days, you develop that action into a habit—whether it is a good action or a bad action. I confess that I don't understand this phenomena of feelings following actions, but from my personal experience, it works.

2. *Don't be ruled by your feelings.* I know my feelings can't be trusted. One minute I feel great and the next minute I'm upset or angry about something or someone. In *My Utmost For His Highest*, Oswald Chambers wrote, "There are certain things in life that we need not pray about—moods, for instance. We will never get rid of moodiness by praying, but we will by kicking it out of our lives. Moods nearly always are rooted in some physical circumstance, not in our true inner self. It is a continual struggle not to listen to the moods which arise as a result of our physical condition, but we must never submit to them for a second. We have to pick ourselves up by the back of the neck and shake ourselves; then we will find that we can do what we believed we were unable to do. The problem that most of us are cursed with is simply that we won't."[2] Recognize the pitfalls of moods and kick yourself into action rather than dwell on the negative sensation.

3. *Ask God to help you.* If you are a person who can't stay motivated no matter how hard you try, then go to God, admit your problem, then ask for His help. I believe one of the main reasons I stay motivated is my belief in God's wonderful plan for my life. I don't want to miss anything that God has planned.

"Wait a minute," you say. "I don't believe that God has a wonderful plan for my life." Then I challenge you to memorize Jeremiah 29:11 and say it every day until you believe in God's plan. It says, ". . . 'For I know the plans I have for you,' declares the LORD, 'plans to prosper you and not to harm you, plans to give you hope and a future.'"

DOWN THE ROAD TOWARD SUCCESS

If you keep a positive motivation, it will send you down the road to success. Some of us have experienced a great deal of success, while

Dig Down Deep—What's Your Motivation?

others aren't very far down the road. It has been said, "Success is a journey and not a destination." Here are some ways to ensure success—not just for First Place, but in life (note the first letter of each paragraph is an acronym for SUCCESS):

S *Set a time each day to be alone with God.* I like the early mornings because they are less hectic. Psalm 63:1 says: "O God, you are my God, earnestly I seek you; my soul thirsts for you, my body longs for you, in a dry and weary land where there is no water."

U *Understand that we have no strength on our own but must depend on God's strength in us.* Isaiah 40:29 says, "He gives strength to the weary and increases the power of the weak."

C *Call on God when fear overtakes your heart.* Psalm 27:1 says: "The LORD is my light and my salvation—whom shall I fear? The LORD is the stronghold of my life—of whom shall I be afraid?"

C *Call on your First Place class members or friends for support and encouragement.* Ecclesiastes 4:12 says: "Though one may be overpowered, two can defend themselves. A cord of three strands is not quickly broken."

E *Enjoy the journey.* Every day is a gift from God and should be celebrated. Psalm 31:24 says: "Be strong and take heart, all you who hope in the LORD."

S *Stay in God's Word each day.* We need that daily turning to God and the Lord can speak to us through His Word, the Bible. Psalm 119:11 says: "I have hidden your word in my heart that I might not sin against you."

S *Seek to love God more today than yesterday.* Our love for our heavenly Father should be increasing each day. John 14:21 says: "Whoever has my commands and obeys them, he is the one who loves me. He who loves me will be loved by my Father, and I too will love him and show myself to him."

I encourage you to memorize each of the above seven verses from the Bible so you can stand against the enemy when you are tempted and he whispers in your ear, "You'll never have success." If you are motivated through the power of God's Spirit, you will arrive at the finish line. Phillipians 1:6 says, "being confident of this, that he who began a good work in you will carry it on to completion until the day of Christ Jesus."

Now that we've stirred your motivation, what sort of obstacles and roadblocks will you have to overcome as you seek to change your lifestyle? We'll examine these roadblocks in the next chapter. Let's turn the page and continue the journey.

CHAPTER FOUR

Obstacles to Overcome

Rhonda Holbrook and her sister, Diana Goodman McDaniel, attended one of our Fitness Week programs several years ago at Ridgecrest Conference Center. Diana, who appeared for five years on the television show *Hee Haw*, had been sent from her church to learn how to begin a First Place program. Rhonda wasn't sure why she was attending. At the time, she weighed 238 pounds. Several months before the Fitness Week, Rhonda had a gall bladder attack. At her doctors' encouragement she eliminated red meat and sugar from her diet and had managed to lose twenty-five pounds. "But I was still overeating," Rhonda says.

After eight hours at the Fitness Week, Rhonda was ready to return home. She had difficulty walking around the conference center. When she called her husband, he said, "Darling, why don't you give it a little more time?" During the second day, we divided into prayer groups, and Rhonda was in my small group. Rhonda thought to herself, *Great, now I'll have to do First Place because I'm in a group with the national director.* As we took prayer requests, Rhonda said, "Carole, I don't know why I'm here this week."

FIRST PLACE

I didn't say anything about her weight but said, "Rhonda, we're glad you've come, and I'm sure God will show you why you are here before the week is over." I didn't know that Rhonda had already tried numerous other programs. She had actually started and stopped one nationally recognized program fifteen times—without success.

The next day during the Bible study session, Rhonda felt the Lord speak to her spirit saying, "When you go back home, Rhonda, I want you to lead the First Place group instead of Diana."

Internally, Rhonda immediately objected and said to the Lord, "I will never be able to take the leadership unless Diana gives me permission without my prompting." After the class, the two sisters left together. When they stepped through the entryway, Diana turned to Rhonda and said, "The Lord has been speaking to my heart. It's not His will for me to lead the First Place group, but He wants you to do it." Rhonda began to cry at the confirmation from God.

The sisters completed the week-long program, returned to their local church, and met with their pastor. While the First Place program does not require that you be at your goal weight to lead a group, Rhonda's pastor objected to Rhonda's leadership, saying, "You have to be an example to lead a weight loss program." The sisters followed their pastor's leadership and instead agreed to begin the thirteen-week study program together. They called each other once a week and followed the other eight commitments of First Place. During the first Bible study, Rhonda found one of her three "life verses"—Romans 12:1: "Therefore, I urge you, brothers, in view of God's mercy, to offer your bodies as living sacrifices, holy and pleasing to God—which is your spiritual worship." Many times in the past, Rhonda had used this verse to present her life to God. She was amazed to see this verse in the first Bible study of First Place. Rhonda got down on her knees and prayed, "God, I can't do this program on my own, but I'm willing to do what You want."

Rhonda and Diana both lost weight during the thirteen weeks. During the first year, Rhonda lost sixty-two pounds and is currently working to lose fifty more pounds through First Place. After the sisters completed their first thirteen-week study, their pastor changed his stance and permitted Rhonda to lead a group at the church. The first session involved twelve ladies; the next had forty men and women. Ultimately the program grew to several groups that totaled about eighty people. As Rhonda considers the benefits she has received from First Place, she says, "I was already a Christian and walking with the Lord, but I didn't allow God to have anything to do with my weight. Now my life is an open book for a fuller, more intimate relationship with Christ."

OBSTACLES TO OVERCOME

Rhonda faced numerous obstacles as she sought to start a First Place program. Your obstacles will be completely different. As you take some initial steps toward a lifestyle change, your mind will cry out with many different excuses. In the next few pages, we'll examine some common obstacles and consider some ways to overcome them. Finally we'll consider the concept of quitting. Many of us have tried numerous weight loss programs in the past. How do you take a proactive stance to prevent quitting again?

"I Don't Have Enough Time."

Time is one of the major excuses used to avoid starting a new program like First Place. You may groan, "I don't have any more hours in my day to exercise or read the Bible. Where will I find the time?"

Each of us has twenty-four hours in a single day. The question is: Do you use that time wisely? The average American spends fifteen hours a week in front of the television set. "Whoa, I don't spend that much time"

FIRST PLACE

you say. One way to judge exactly how much time you spend at the television set is to keep track for a few days. The results may surprise you. We rationalize television because of our love for sports or the need to follow the news, yet it takes up a lot of time. You can free up a few more hours in your day if you simply turn off the television set.

Another way to gain more time each day is to set the alarm clock a half hour or an hour earlier. Then use that extra time in a productive fashion. Monday through Friday, I don my exercise clothes and work out with friends before work. I eliminate the excuse of no time by planning this activity into my schedule.

God created everything in the world, including time. He has the hours of the day for our schedule—particularly as we turn over those hours into His hands. Solomon wrote about God in the early pages of Ecclesiastes 3:11, saying: "He has made everything beautiful in its time. He has also set eternity in the hearts of men; yet they cannot fathom what God has done from beginning to end." Also the psalmist says, "This is the day the LORD has made; let us rejoice and be glad in it" (Psalm 118:24). Finally, the apostle Paul encourages us to make good use of our time because the days are evil (Ephesians 5:16).

"I'll Never Be Able to Do It."

Sometimes we look at ourselves and hear a little voice inside that says, "You are a loser. You will never be able to take off those pounds." This kind of self-talk may have started as a small child when someone in school called you "stupid." Instead of responding with a "Forrest Gump" sort of answer ("Stupid is as stupid does"), you took that message to heart and began to call yourself names. These names and self-talk become another obstacle in your goal to lose weight and change your lifestyle.

If you have these negative messages spinning in your head (and many of us do), I hope you will open your Bible and remind yourself of God's great love for you. The Lord told the prophet Jeremiah in 31:3, "The LORD appeared to us in the past, saying: 'I have loved you with an everlasting love; I have drawn you with loving-kindness.'"

Obstacles to Overcome

This truth is only one of the many precious thoughts from God's Word. We need to hold onto these verses when we feel something inside tell us that we are not able to do the First Place program or when we face any other obstacle.

"I Don't Have the Discipline."

Sometimes we chafe at the disciplines involved with First Place. You may look at the nine commitments and instantly conclude, "I don't have the discipline. I admit that I don't have what it takes."

Within the First Place program, you are not alone. As part of a small group, you have other members in your group who can help encourage the different disciplines, such as reading your Bible, doing your Fact Sheet, or making your weekly phone call. Or, if you're doing the First Place program with two or three friends, mutual support is going to help you persevere. Many First Place members find it especially difficult to make this weekly phone call. As a society, we've built relational walls around ourselves to keep people from hurting us because we've been rejected and hurt many times in the past. Through First Place, God wants to bring emotional healing and encourage you in this particular discipline.

Why do we reach out to other people within First Place? Because we learn to love other people with the love that God has shown to us through Christ. I grew up in a generation that said, "If people don't conform to what we tell them to do, then let's just forget about them." Through reading the Bible, I've learned that God has a totally different perspective. He says that He loves every individual as much as He loves you and me. It is unimportant what they've done or what kind of sin they have committed. In God's eyes, there are no degrees of sin. However, sin separates us from God. In 1 John 1:9–10 God's Word says: "If we confess our sins, he is faithful and just and will forgive us our sins and purify us from all unrighteousness. If we claim we have not sinned, we make him out to be a liar and his word has no place in our lives." When we fail and miss a particular discipline, then we turn to God, ask His forgiveness, and try again.

FIRST PLACE

We will not pretend that discipline is easy. It takes a certain type of discipline to attend a weekly meeting, to fill out the Fact Sheet with what you eat, and to have regular Bible study. Each of these commitments involves discipline. But what are the results of discipline? Hebrews 12:11 says, "No discipline seems pleasant at the time, but painful. Later on, however, it produces a harvest of righteousness and peace for those who have been trained by it." If you want a harvest of righteousness and peace, then you must follow the course of discipline.

"I'm Afraid I Will Fail."

Fear is a universal problem. It weakens our hearts, robs us of peace of mind, and saps our energy. Unfortunately, fear is alive and well in the world of weight loss. Many people are afraid they will fail again after so many previous attempts to lose weight. After they have been in First Place and have reached their weight goal, some people are afraid they will gain back their weight. Also, leaders of First Place groups are afraid they won't be effective and that members of the group will drop out of the program.

In the Bible, the admonition to "fear not" is used more than a hundred times. God knows us well enough to know that we need constant reminders to live in trust and dependence on Him rather than living in fear and anxiety. I have found several things to be true for my own life when fears overtake me. Here are four steps to help you overcome your fears:

1. Choose to obey God and leave the consequences of life to Him. Joshua 22:5 says: "But be very careful to . . . love the LORD your God, to walk in all his ways, to obey his commands, to hold fast to him and to serve him with all your heart and all your soul."
2. Recognize that God is greater than your circumstances. Romans 8:31 says, "What, then, shall we say in response to this? If God is for us, who can be against us?"
3. Ask God to make you aware of His presence. In Isaiah 41:10, the prophet wrote, "So do not fear, for I am with you. . . . I will

strengthen you and help you; I will uphold you with my righteous right hand."

4. Praise God for delivering you from your fears. Psalm 34:1, 4 says: "I will extol the LORD at all times; his praise will always be on my lips. . . . I sought the LORD, and he answered me; he delivered me from all my fears."

Take these four steps into your life and heart as you seek to conquer the obstacle of fear in your life, whether it concerns weight loss or anything else you encounter.

NO MATTER WHAT THE OBSTACLE—DON'T QUIT

Some of you today feel like you want to quit. In your mind, you have failed with your weight, and you wonder how you will be able to restore the years ahead. I love the section of the Old Testament where the nation of Israel has sunk low in the eyes of the world. The prophet Joel reminds them about how God will bring restoration, saying: "I will repay you for the years the locusts have eaten. . . . You will have plenty to eat, until you are full, and you will praise the name of the LORD your God, who has worked wonders for you" (Joel 2:25, 26). We need to develop consistency so we don't quit.

So many times, I say to our heavenly Father, "I'm in way over my head, Lord. This is too big. When you called me to be involved in First Place, you never told me it was going to be like this." In my own mind, I try to have a pity party with God. Perhaps you've done the same thing with your weight or your relationship to God—you feel like quitting.

Then, once again, God reassures me that there is nothing I can't do if He is doing it through me. I must refocus away from quitting and focus on the God of the impossible. He doesn't want me to quit.

One day I heard Ann Landers discuss the results of a survey among parents. To my surprise, many of the parents said that if they had it to do over again, they would never have had children. Those parents wanted to quit, and that attitude is symptomatic of the world that we live in.

Some people say that their reason for quitting is laziness. A lot of times we are lazy about our habits and lifestyle. We tire of doing everything right all the time. Sure we get tired of filling out the Fact Sheet and eating all the right foods, but it's not laziness that stops us. It's fear. Underneath everything we are afraid that if we commit to the First Place program and fail, then people will think less about God. Is God's reputation at stake when we quit? No. God will still be God. Besides, the success is not in the program itself but in the process. The success of the program is a continual dependence on God. We need to give Him First Place in our every decision; then in His power we will be able to conquer our fears and concerns.

If fear makes us want to quit, then where does fear come from? Satan is definitely the author of fear. First Peter 5:8 in the Living Bible says: "Be careful. Watch out for attacks from Satan your great enemy. He prowls around like a hungry roaring lion looking for some victim to tear apart." Notice that the Bible doesn't say that Satan *is* a lion—only that he acts like one. Let's look at some of the characteristics of a lion. First, lions chase away their own young. In the same way, many of us have been chased away from God before we were fully mature. God wants us to mature in our relationship with Him. This can happen through the First Place program; I've seen it happen in many different people.

Second, a lion attacks sick, young, or straggling animals. The enemy knows when we are at our weakest point, so he attacks. When it comes to weight loss, Satan may be whispering to you, "You knew you could never succeed in this program. Why look: you lost thirty pounds then gained back ten. Why not just quit?" The temptation is there to quit the program. However, Matthew 4:23 tells us that Jesus Christ went about healing the sick. If you feel weak or sick, then turn to Jesus; He is strong when we are weak. I draw great encouragement from the passage about Jesus that says: "For we do not have a high priest who is unable to sympathize with our weaknesses, but we have one who has

Obstacles to Overcome

been tempted in every way, just as we are—yet was without sin" (Hebrews 4:15).

The third characteristic of lions is that they choose victims who are alone or not alert. In my own life, I know it is not good for me to be alone. For that reason, I don't keep any food in my home that is not a part of the First Place program. This means that I don't keep any cookies or sweets. It may be a step of protection that you will also need to take in your own home. As the First Place national director, I'm not going to eat anything in front of you that you shouldn't eat. This means that I will not let my husband purchase boxes of Girl Scout cookies and slip them into our freezer. I know if those cookies are in my freezer and I'm alone in my home, then Satan will begin to attack. I may deflect the first wave of the attack—determined that I'm not going to give in to those cookies. But if I'm left alone long enough, I'll eat the cookies. I know myself well enough to know that I don't need to be alone with foods that I can't have. You too will need to consider this type of obstacle in your own life and make some choices about it.

It is important to remember that if you have a personal relationship with Jesus Christ, you are never alone. Jesus says in Hebrews 13:5, "Never will I leave you; never will I forsake you." Satan makes us feel alone, but Jesus is our Comforter. When you feel alone, run to Jesus.

The fourth characteristic of a lion is that it hunts at night. The lion is a cowardly creature to need the cover of darkness. In the same way, Satan attacks us at night because that's when we are the most vulnerable. We may be tired or sleepy, and our thinking is not as sharp as in the morning when we are refreshed and geared up for the day ahead. Several years ago I took a good friend to a conference, and she received tremendous emotional healing in her life. The night was usually a difficult time for her, but one morning she came to my hotel room with her face glowing. During the night she had latched onto a verse from Psalm 139:12: "Even the darkness will not be dark to you; the night will shine like the day." The daytime and the nighttime are the same to God. We need to stay in the light and run from the darkness.

FIRST PLACE

Finally, a lion patiently stalks its prey with a short, rapid charge. Satan is patient with me and knows how to work on my mind. I used to have a real weakness for Baskin-Robbins ice cream and there was a shop right down the street from my house. If I went somewhere, I headed down that particular street—whether I had any business there or not. In fact, if I was anywhere near that street, I turned and got on the street that ran past Baskin-Robbins. Before long I would tell myself, "Well, I don't have to stop." Then my tune changed to, "I may or I may not stop." In reality, I had already made a decision and it was done: I was stopping at Baskin-Robbins. Because I entertained the thought, the fact had been completed. Our pastor, in a sermon on temptation, summarized the process, saying, "Temptation; hesitation; participation."

Although your particular weakness will be different than mine, you need to turn control of your weaknesses over into God's capable hands.

Yes, there are many times when I face an obstacle in my weight loss program. I feel like quitting. Patsy Clairmont told the story about her little boy at about age six. She walked with him down to the bus stop since they lived out in the country. She said before she got back to the house, her son had beat her home. She said to him, "What in the world are you doing? The school bus is coming soon."

He looked her straight in the eye and said firmly, "I'm quitting school."

With determination in her eyes, she said, "You can't quit school, and besides, you are only in the first grade. Why are you quitting?"

The boy looked down at the ground and said, "Well, it's too long, it's too hard, and it's boring."

She said, "Son, that's life. Get on the bus."[1]

Sometimes I have to tell this little story to myself. I have to say, "Carole, this is life. Get on the bus." God didn't promise us that life would be rosy and without difficulty. Instead, the Lord promised to carry us through any situation and any trial. Romans 8:28 says, "And we know that in all things God works for the good of those who love him, who have been called according to his purpose."

Obstacles to Overcome

As you read about First Place in this book, God knows the obstacles and excuses that you will mount to try and quit. But quitting isn't the answer. Instead, you need to cling even tighter to the hand of God and ask for His strength and enabling in order to walk another step along the journey. He is more than able to accomplish what concerns you today.

In the next chapter, we'll dig deeper into what the Scriptures say about what we eat and our need to be in balance. This spiritual discipline has some unique aspects.

Let's turn the page and continue our journey to Christ-centered health.

CHAPTER FIVE

The Spiritual Foundation

One of Roberta Wasserman's most painful childhood memories involved her weight. In elementary school, every student was herded through a physical. Everyone stood on weight scales in the middle of the gym. When Roberta stepped on the scale, the needle moved past the 100-pound mark. Devastated in front of her peers, Roberta internalized the humiliation of that moment. Her mother took Roberta to Weight Watchers and she lost weight but began many years of self-abuse.

"My weight yo-yoed through my teens," she says, "One small bite of food made me feel too fat and the distorted body image I saw was unacceptable. Then the deprivation eventually led me to overeat where a thousand bites were not enough." Attending a meeting of Overeater's Anonymous, the other women were shocked that Roberta would attend because she was so "tiny." They were unaware of her struggle with bulimia.

Through Christian therapy, Roberta got in touch with the sad, wounded side of her life and found help for her bulimia disorder. Because she wanted to lose forty pounds, Roberta joined a First Place group at a local church near her home in Riva, Maryland. Roberta was Christian, but her spiritual life took a huge jump through First Place. She says, "First Place got me in touch with the source of the Healer of my wounds, my Lord and Savior Jesus Christ. For the first time in my life, I began to write my daily prayers. I read the Bible and the Scriptures came to life."

While in First Place, Roberta lost about forty pounds and today she continues in an accountable relationship to several group members and keeps the nine commitments. "I've spent a lifetime turning to food, my false god. With the help of First Place, I've gradually come to realize that I can stare at my open pantry and know there will never be enough food to satisfy my soul because only the Lord can meet that need." In First Place, Roberta has gained a treasured relationship with Jesus Christ.

BACK TO BASICS

Three years ago I had a bulging disc in my neck. This physical ailment returned me to the basics in my emotional, mental, physical, and spiritual life. My hurting neck landed me in bed for several weeks and finally in physical therapy.

For many years, I had resisted any sort of weight training. When I started the First Place program, I began to walk, then jog. I loved jogging but I despised strapping into a weight machine and lifting weights. Yet the physical therapy for my neck involved weights. After several weeks of therapy, I said, "Hey, I don't need to pay you to do these exercises. We've got the same machines at our church workout room, and I can do it on my own."

For years, people had seen me jogging on the track at our church with friends, and one man in particular had been encouraging me to lift weights. I never made any pretense about lifting weights; I was *not* going to start it. When this man saw me begin in the weight room after my neck injury, he laughed, saying, "Carole, I've been after you

The Spiritual Foundation

for three years to work on your upper body." It took my neck pain to return me to the basics. I now know that as long as I exercise and lift weights, I don't have any pain. But if I quit my exercises for a week or two, then the pain returns in my neck. I have to stick with the basics.

I'm one of the few people you will meet who absolutely loves to exercise. Several years ago my husband, Johnny, and I went to the Smokey Mountains for a week. We loved the gorgeous October weather and enjoyed hiking in the forests as the leaves were turning their brilliant colors. One morning we packed a lunch and hiked two and a half miles each direction to a waterfall. On the way up to the waterfall, I crossed a small bridge and the bottom step was wet. My tennis shoe turned and my foot twisted, tearing some ligaments in my ankle. My injury was made worse because I had to walk over two miles to get assistance. The injury put a halt to my jogging for six months. After not jogging for six months, it was like starting over again—I had to return to the basics. Although I bristle when I have to begin again, this is a very real part of life.

One of my friends, Chris, saw my reaction at starting over and said, "Carole, starting over is a basic part of any recovery. In Alcoholics Anonymous they tell you to take one day at a time." When you, the reader, look at your weight situation, you may feel totally out of control. You need to return to the basics in order to understand your spiritual foundation. In the pages that follow, we will examine what the Bible has to say about our bodies, what we eat, how to achieve balance, and the consequences of disobedience. Finally we will look at three aspects of returning to the basics.

BIBLICAL BASICS

The First Place program isn't built on a theory or a premise but on the solid truth that has stood the test of the ages—the Bible. The Bible says a great deal about everything in life. Its pages are inspired and have the absolute authority to teach us how to live to the fullest.

FIRST PLACE

Before we examine First Place in detail, let's consider what God says about His plan and desires.

First, when it comes to the physical aspects of life, our bodies are the temple of the Holy Spirit. If you have asked Jesus Christ to come into your life as your Savior, then God's Spirit lives in you. Paul reminded the church at Corinth about this fact when he said, "Do you not know that your body is the temple of the Holy Spirit, who is in you, whom you have received from God? You are not your own; you were bought at a price. Therefore honor God with your body" (1 Cor. 6:19–20). It is our spiritual obligation to honor God with our physical bodies. You may not like the current shape of your physical body; that is why you have turned to First Place. As you follow the First Place program, you are improving your physical temple where God's Spirit lives. You can feel good about the fact that you are improving your body.

Balance and moderation are also basic spiritual tenants that are reinforced repeatedly in the Scriptures. Consider for a moment the life of the Lord Jesus when He walked the face of the earth. The apostle Luke tells us in Luke 2:52: "So Jesus grew both tall [physical] and wise [mental], and was loved by God [spiritual] and man [emotional]" (LB). Jesus had a sense of balance in His life. Yet besides the example of Christ's life, He also encouraged us to have balance. When Jesus was asked about the greatest commandment for man, He said, "'Love the Lord your God with all your heart [emotional] and with all your soul [spiritual] and with all your strength [physical] and with all your mind' [mental]; and, 'Love your neighbor as yourself'" (Luke 10:27).

Besides balance, the Scriptures also exhort us to live in moderation. Overeating, overdrinking, or any type of excessive behavior is not pleasing to God. Paul wrote the church, saying: "Let your moderation be known unto all men. The Lord is at hand" (Phil. 4:5, KJV).

If we obey God's desire for our life and maintain a sense of balance, then we can enjoy the spiritual, emotional, mental, and physical blessings of God. God honors our obedience with His blessing. As the psalmist wrote in Psalm 103:2–5: "Praise the LORD, O my soul, and

The Spiritual Foundation

forget not all his benefits. He forgives all my sins and heals all my diseases; he redeems my life from the pit and crowns me with love and compassion. He satisfies my desires with good things, so that my youth is renewed like the eagle's."

These words of the psalm encourage us to celebrate God's benefits and to obey the words of Scripture. Isaiah tells us that we will have peace from God as we follow the Scriptures: "This is what the LORD says—your Redeemer, the Holy One of Israel: 'I am the LORD your God, who teaches you what is best for you, who directs you in the way you should go. If only you had paid attention to my commands, your peace would have been like a river, your righteousness like the waves of the sea" (Isa. 48:17–18).

The Bible even has a few words of wisdom about too much food consumption: "When you sit to dine with a ruler, note well what is before you, and put a knife to your throat if you are given to gluttony. Do not crave his delicacies, for that food is deceptive. . . . For drunkards and gluttons become poor, and drowsiness clothes them in rags. (Pro. 23:1–3, 21).

WHY DO WE RETURN TO THE BASICS?

It's tiresome to keep going back to the basics. In First Place, we are always starting over again. Before I know it, it's time to join another thirteen-week group. Maybe you joined a group and didn't find any success during those thirteen weeks. Why do it again? For me, the reason to repeat is found in Romans 8:29, where Paul writes, "For those God foreknew he also predestined to be conformed to the likeness of his Son, that he might be the firstborn among many brothers." God has a purpose when we have to start over again. That purpose is to cause us to look more like His Son, Jesus Christ. As we return to the basics, then God can mold us into the person that He wants.

The woodcarver looks at a block of wood and sees a beautiful, carved wooden duck inside that block. God looks at our outside and sees that through the carving process we too can be a beautiful creation. It's like God says to us, "If you will not quit, then I will do My work in your life." In the First Place program, success is found in the process or the journey.

There are three basics that will take you into a deeper relationship with God and Jesus Christ. *First, you need to start First Place.* Our own office staff participates in the thirteen-week First Place program. This last session they lost a total of 121 pounds and everyone turned in a Fact Sheet every week. We stayed on the Live-It program every week and each of us lost weight. Is it amazing? No, we know our program works, and it works because in the process, God blesses us with success. Although we sometimes want someone else to do the work, only we can do the work of First Place. It can't be done by anyone else. Even our staff knows the value of starting over. God is the God of "beginning again."

When my ankle was hurt, a stationary bike was all I could do to continue my exercise program. Some mornings I would wake up and think, *I don't want to get on that stationary bike for my exercise. In fact, I hate that thing because it doesn't go anywhere and I have to just sit there.* Still I had to begin again.

For me, exercise is an appointment that I made more than thirteen years ago, and I still show up for that appointment five times each week. When I'm at home, I go down to the track at the church and exercise with my friends. If I'm not there, people will ask me, "What happened to you today, Carole?" Of course, I don't always feel like going; but when I show up, God always meets me there. Invariably on some of my worst days, I'll be jogging along and somebody will show up that I have not seen in a long time. We will jog together and begin sharing what the Lord has done in our lives. The exercise time flies by; I don't want it to end because I know that the Lord brought that particular person that day.

I've always got plenty of excuses when it comes to not exercising. However, I've found that when I feel sluggish and not anxious to exercise, that's when I must push myself out to go ahead and do it anyway.

The Spiritual Foundation

Somewhere along the way, my attitude changes and the exercise becomes enjoyable. Zig Ziglar says that if you want anything to become a habit, you need to do it for at least twenty-one days without missing a day.[1]

People have told me how they had exercised regularly for three years, then they suddenly quit for two weeks because of sickness or some other illness. Before they knew it, a year had passed without regular exercise. Bad habits are easy to accumulate, but they too can be broken with a fresh start.

One of the commitments in First Place is to fill out a Fact Sheet with all of the food that you have eaten. I've been filling out a Fact Sheet since 1981. Sometimes I go through this mental process: "This isn't so bad. I can have that type of food if I want. I'll cut back a little bit later." Or I say, "I've had a hard day and I need to eat this. I'll do better tomorrow." If I continue to go down the road with this kind of thinking, what happens? One bad day gets added to another bad day. That is why in the First Place program if you eat something that is not on the program—like a candy bar or a piece of pie (anything with sugar in it)—you put that item on the back of your Fact Sheet. Then for your next meal, you start again on the First Place program. You forget about the food on the back and eat good nutrition the next meal. When you do this, your mind and your emotions acknowledge that you made an unwise choice for weight loss, but you begin all over again the very next meal. You want to avoid saying, "Oh, I ate something that I wasn't supposed to eat. I'll skip my next meal and do better tonight." That way of thinking will lead to binging by nightfall. Then after binging, you'll believe you've blown the program for the entire week and tailspin into a major stall. Remember, the first basic principle is to always begin again.

The second basic principle is to *learn how to fail*. Some of us do not know how to fail gracefully. You have to be willing to risk failure if you are going to do anything significant in life. Thomas Edison failed thousands of times before he invented the electric light bulb. I can't see many of us failing thousands of times before we quit. Instead we would chalk it up, saying, "Well, that just isn't meant to be." Someone once asked Thomas Edison about all of his failures, and he said, "I have learned a lot of ways *not* to do something."

Tim Hansel, in his book *Holy Sweat*, tells the story of a young man starting his job as a new president of a bank. The new president went to the retiring president and said, "I need to ask you a question."

The older distinguished gentleman looked up and the younger man asked, "What it is that makes you a success?"

The man smiled and said, "Two words—*good decisions*."

The young man said, "Oh, thank you." And he walked out of the room, but in a minute he came back puzzled and said, "Sir, I need to ask another question. How do you make good decisions?"

The older gentleman looked up from his desk and said, "One word—*experience*."

"Oh, thank you, sir," said the young man and walked out of the room, but almost immediately he returned.

The older bank president put his pen down and looked up. The younger man asked, "How do you get that experience?"

"Two words—*bad decisions*."[2]

In my life, I have learned some of my most valuable lessons from bad decisions. Don't be afraid of failing. If you are afraid to fail, you will miss some of the most valuable lessons of life. Paul talked about this process in Romans 7:19-20: "For what I do is not the good I want to do; no, the evil I do not want to do—this I keep on doing. Now if I do what I do not want to do, it is no longer I who do it, but it is sin living in me that does it." Many times we fail because of sin in our life but God takes us right back through that failure to teach us lessons that would not be learned through any other manner.

God gives us a lot of rope in our lives. Although I deserve a lot of judgment from God, He continually shows me mercy. He gives me a long rope but eventually pulls it in saying, "Are you convinced now that you cannot do a better job than I can do?" God knows that we must realize our failures so we will lean more heavily on His power in our lives.

The Spiritual Foundation

In the area of weight loss, you may have failed many times. Give that failure into God's hands, saying, "I have proven to You that I'm a failure. I cannot do this. I cannot lose weight. Even if I do lose weight, I always gain it back. I'm a failure." The Lord has been waiting for you to reach this decision point, and He will respond, "You are not going to be a failure anymore; because if you let me do it, I'll do it." Through the commitments in First Place, we learn that failure is never fatal. We also learn that when we do fail, we simply give that failure to God and begin again.

The third and final basic point is to *persevere*. The apostle Paul knew about perseverance and wrote the Philippian church, saying, "I press on toward the goal to win the prize for which God has called me heavenward in Christ Jesus" (Phil. 3:14). Paul exhorted us to keep moving toward our goals despite any obstacles we might experience.

Have you ever prayed for patience? The Bible tells us that we get patience through tribulation. Sometimes I'd like to ignore Romans 5:3 which says: "We can rejoice, too, when we run into problems and trials [and everyone has problems and trials], for we know that they are good for us—they help us learn to be patient" (LB). That Scripture alone is enough to convince me never to *pray* for patience. I've got enough problems and trials in my life without asking God to send more. Instead, we need to learn how to persevere, because perseverance is patience plus endurance.

Also, perseverance is a gift from God that reminds us of our options. Yes, we can quit. I've quit for months at a time, but God always draws me back. Many times I want to quit when the Holy Spirit is dealing with an area of my life that I am unwilling to change. I don't want to deal with it, so I draw back. In fact, I've sometimes done this for as long as six weeks, but God keeps after me to return. When I finally return to God's everlasting arms, I think, "Why did I waste six weeks?" Those feelings of peace don't come until I obey with my mind and my will. As I said in an earlier chapter, actions never follow feelings, but feelings always follow actions. Perseverance has nothing to do with feelings but everything to do with our continual relationship with Jesus Christ.

FIRST PLACE

Tim Hansel included the following poem by Philip Brewer in his book, *Holy Sweat*:[3]

The Paradoxes of Man

Strong enough to be weak.
Successful enough to fail.
Busy enough to take time.
Wise enough to say, "I don't know."
Serious enough to laugh.
Rich enough to be poor.
Right enough to say, "I'm wrong."
Compassionate enough to
   discipline.
Conservative enough to give freely.
Mature enough to be childlike.
Righteous enough to be a sinner.
Important enough to be last.
Courageous enough to fear God.
Planned enough to be spontaneous.
Controlled enough to be flexible.
Free enough to endure captivity.
Knowledgeable enough to ask
   questions.
Loving enough to be angry.
Great enough to be anonymous.
Responsible enough to play.
Assured enough to be rejected.
Stable enough to cry.
Victorious enough to lose.
Industrious enough to relax.
Leading enough to serve.

The Bible is full of paradoxes. Jesus says that if you want to have something, then you have to give it away. If you want to be strong, then you

The Spiritual Foundation

have to be weak. If we want to find the Scriptural foundation for our Christ-centered health program, then we need to return to the basics. We must begin again, learn to fail, and never give up.

One of the keys to First Place is finding balance. We explore this concept in the next chapter.

CHAPTER SIX

Discovering Balance

For more than twenty years Terry Dollar, from Marion, Indiana, was overweight and could feel her emotions spiraling out of control. By the end of 1995, the doctor gave Terry a diagnosis of severe depression and anxiety. The next month her depression increased because her grandmother died and her only sister, Becky's, chemotherapy was not working. Because of her poor concentration, Terry lost her job and began caring for her sister. Terry's eating habits came into focus on Valentine's Day at Becky's home. Terry finished off a pound box of chocolate and was almost unaware that she had eaten it. Becky became upset, and in a dying wish, asked her sister to lose weight. Terry lost her sister to cancer on February 23.

Later that spring a First Place program was started at her church, and Terry joined the group. At the first meeting she weighed in at 284 pounds, almost twice what her 5-foot, 8-inch frame should carry. After a year in the program, Terry lost 133 pounds and is within ten pounds of her goal weight. Yet from her perspective, First Place has done much more than help her achieve weight loss.

Twenty-five years earlier Terry had become a Christian, but she had never in any real sense turned control of her life

FIRST PLACE

over to Jesus. Before starting First Place, Terry vowed never to diet again because it was too difficult and she always gained back more than she lost. She says, "For Becky's sake, I gave First Place the last chance and told the Lord, 'I know my weight is a poor witness for You; it's killing my knees and most likely me. So if it's Your will that I lose weight, You'll have to do the bulk of the work. I turn it all over to You.'"

God honored Terry's sincere prayer and took over. Since her involvement in the First Place program, her depression is gone, she has more energy, and her knees don't hurt. Terry explains the changes in her life saying, "He has given me a stronger faith in Him, and I have truly given Him first place in my life. I know Becky is in heaven with God cheering me on."

LIFE OUT OF CONTROL

Sometimes our lives whirl out of control. In your life, perhaps your consumption of food is out of control. Or possibly a relationship has suddenly been broken in your family or among your friends. Maybe your work has piled so high that it is out of control. For many years, I loved reading good novels, and this area of my life got out of control. In the early 80s, my mother took my sister and me on a trip through Austria. I had never been to that part of the world. At the airport, before boarding the plane, our minister of music, who was traveling with us, recommended that I buy a copy of *The Thornbirds* to read during the trip. While traveling through some of the most panoramic scenery in the world, I had my eyes glued to the printed page of that novel. I read that thick book in the back of the bus throughout Austria. Occasionally I would stray from my novel when someone said, "Oh, that's beautiful." I looked out the windows, saw it quickly, and returned to my novel. My reading habits had whirled out of control, and I was stuck in *The Thornbirds* while missing Austria.

Discovering Balance

Other times my life gets out of control in the area of relationships. Sometimes things start out right, then turn upside down. A while back we eliminated cable television from our home. We had the basic cable and determined that for the money, it cost too much and should be eliminated—even the minimum service. Our lack of cable television posed a bit of a problem for my husband (who decided to get rid of it). Johnny has never been a good sleeper, and when he wakes up in the middle of the night and has trouble sleeping, he turns on the television. We laughed about taking away his pacifier.

The next morning when I kissed him goodbye, I asked, "Did you sleep well?"

He smiled and said, "I really did sleep well last night."

The truth was, I had slept well for the first time in quite a while because Johnny wasn't up watching television throughout the night. As I left for work, I had a warm feeling toward Johnny. After several hours in my office, I thought I would call him just to chat. On our phone, we have call waiting and Johnny hates to use this convenience. When I called he was on the phone, and it took about eight rings on his end to answer it. With every single ring, Johnny grew more uptight hearing the beep on his end. Finally he managed to push the right button and said an exasperated, "Hello."

I said, in a cheery voice, "Just me."

He abruptly said, "Well, I'll have to call you back, I'm on the other line." He hung up, and I stepped out of my office to get an apple. While I was gone, Johnny called me back. My assistant said, "She'll be back in a few minutes."

When Johnny called back a second time, he said, "Well, what did you want? I was on the phone." Well, you know that warm feeling that I had a few minutes earlier? It evaporated.

I said to him, "I didn't really want anything in particular. I just wanted to see how you were doing. You know we didn't get to talk much this morning." After a few more minutes, our conversation ended. My warm feeling for Johnny had disappeared, and I wanted that feeling back instead of the confusion. It seemed like the circumstances of my day were going into a tailspin. What had started as a warm fuzzy had ended as a cold lumpy.

When I feel like things are spiraling downward in my life and circumstances, God has taught me that whether I'm right side up or upside down, I need to turn those circumstances over to Him. He is the only one who can bring balance into my life when it is unbalanced.

BALANCE IN EVERY ASPECT OF LIFE

The First Place program is designed to bring balance to every area of life: mental, physical, spiritual, and emotional. Since the First Place food plan is not a diet but a way of life, we encourage every participant to begin with a willingness to change his or her lifestyle in a variety of areas for balance and personal growth. We accomplish this lifestyle change through completing, to the best of our ability, the nine commitments that are detailed in the next two chapters. Most of us will not be able to accomplish every one of the nine commitments every day. Nonetheless, we strive for this goal because, if reached, it will bring balance to our lives. Our heavenly Father has a single-minded purpose: to conform us to the image of His son, Jesus. In the New Living Translation, Romans 8:29 says, "For God knew his people in advance, and he chose them to become like his Son, so that his Son would be the firstborn, with many brothers and sisters." Did you catch the significance of that verse? God selected us to become like Jesus. For this process to take place, God wants to change us in every area of life.

Through First Place you will be involved in a plan that incorporates the four major areas of life: mental, physical, emotional, and spiritual. The changes in each area of your life can be quite dramatic. Frequently I meet men and women who initially joined the First Place program with weight loss as their main goal. After they reach their weight loss goal, these same people say the spiritual changes have been the most significant changes in their life. As God receives His rightful position in our lives, many unexpected blessings occur. Matthew 6:33

Discovering Balance

tells us: "Seek ye first the kingdom of God, and his righteousness, and all these things shall be added unto you" (KJV). In the pages that follow, we will examine each of the four areas and explore why balance is important in each one.

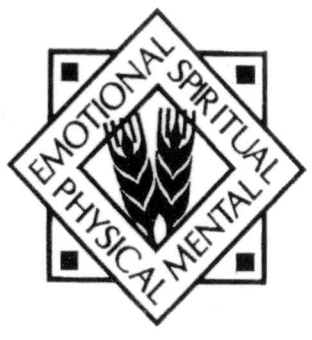

MENTAL

"Do not conform any longer to the pattern of this world, but be transformed by the renewing of your mind. Then you will be able to test and approve what God's will is—His good, pleasing and perfect will" (Rom. 12:2).

For most of us, when it comes to using our mind, we are just plain lazy. We only use a fraction of the mental capacities that God has given us. As we grow older, if we don't stay mentally active, we begin to lose brain power.

In First Place, we are challenged to think and use our mental capabilities in several ways.

Learn Scripture

Each week we memorize one verse of Scripture and recite it when we weigh in at our meeting. I encourage you to practice this memory verse with a friend or family member if you are not participating in a group. Initially you may scoff at memorizing a single verse from the Bible. If you stay in the program for one year, you will have memorized forty Bible verses, one for each week of four ten-week Bible studies. In First Place we also read and study our Bibles, then discuss our Bible study at our weekly meeting. I have found that if I don't have a regular Bible study in a group, then I tend to grow lax when I study on my own initiative. Last summer, because of my intense travel schedule, I wasn't in a regular study group. I decided to be independent and purchase a Kay Arthur Bible study at my Christian book store so I could study on my own. At the end of the summer, I had not completed the first week. I believe each of us is more effective when we are accountable to others in some sort of a small group.

Use Your "Dead Time"

Maybe you don't feel like you have any "dead time" but each of us has some space in our day that has nothing going on—for example, in the car, waiting in a doctor's office, or standing in line at the supermarket. In First Place, we use these empty moments to listen, read, memorize, or study. In the Houston area, we have a lot of "dead time" driving across town because of frequent traffic jams. In 1985, I decided that I needed to fill this time with things of God, and audiotapes appeared to be a perfect solution. However, tapes of Scripture, Christian music, or motivational talks were not a luxury I felt that I could afford at that time. I mentioned the idea in my First Place meeting, and the next week, a woman in my class arrived with a grocery bag full of tapes. She explained: "I want you to have these tapes. My husband and I have been to every seminar that comes to town. These tapes are from motivational speakers, and I don't need you to return them. Please listen to them; then give them to others." I followed her advice and still listen to tapes of sermons or motivational talks when I exercise or drive in my car. You can use this method to stimulate your own mental activity. At first, it may seem hard; but as you practice, it becomes a way of life. I have found that the more I know and learn, the more my desire to know and learn grows.

Avoid Negative Thinking

I believe that the mind is the most significant player in our quest for emotional stability. A number of people who enter the First Place

Discovering Balance

program suffer from emotional abuse, both from others in the past and also from negative thinking that they heap on themselves. Zig Ziglar calls this "stinkin' thinkin'." Do you have these sorts of mental messages in your mind?

They could be something like, *I'll never lose that weight. It took me years to get here. I've lost a few pounds before and gained it right back. Why will this be different?*

Or perhaps you tell yourself, *See how stupid that sounded. I'm not even capable of putting together a coherent sentence. What business do I have saying anything in a small group?* Your particular messages may be completely different, but whatever they are, they spring into your mind uninvited. Whenever you have a bad week, this negative thinking overtakes your emotions and you come to class feeling hopeless and depressed. No one is immune; it can happen to participants and leaders alike.

In June 1997, I had shoulder surgery; for six weeks my only exercise was during my physical therapy sessions three times a week. In my mind, I rationalized that a regular workout schedule was impossible, so I planned to wait until my therapy concluded before starting my regular exercise again. Actually, I *had* exercised during this six-week period at the two First Place Fitness Weeks at Ridgecrest and Glorieta conference centers. I thought I needed to be a role model for our participants in the area of exercise. Still, my mind had just convinced my emotions that it would be better to wait until I *felt* like exercising voluntarily before I resumed my regular exercise schedule.

During this time I went through a sort of transformation in this area of my life. I began to dwell on the aches and pains of my shoulder until I was depressed. Hopeless feelings washed over me; I thought I would never be whole again. One Monday, after several weeks of my strange behavior, my assistant, Pat Lewis, said to me, "Carole, is something else wrong, or is it just your shoulder bothering you?"

Quickly I answered, "Nothing else is wrong, Pat. It's just my shoulder." Yet I continued to think about her question all afternoon. As I thought about it, I understood that my physical condition was consuming my thoughts—day and night. During the night hours, I hadn't been able to sleep well because I woke up every time I turned over. During the day, I constantly assessed my physical condition: was it better, or worse? Suddenly I understood that because I had given up my exercise routine, the balance of my life had become upset.

The next morning I began my normal presurgery routine. I got up, had my quiet time, and left home so I arrived at the gym by 6:00 A.M. I had a great workout and, to my amazement, a wonderful day. For the first time in six weeks, I felt energized and enthusiastic. My newfound knowledge about myself brought such excitement that on Wednesday I went to the gym at 5:30 A.M. so I could keep my 7:15 physical therapy appointment. I felt my therapy would go better than it had in the past. And I was right. I walked into the session, and when asked, "How are you feeling?" I said "Great," instead of my usual, "Oh, maybe a little better." Everything looked different and brighter than it had on Monday. What was the difference?

Nothing radical had changed with my shoulder; it still needed time to heal. The difference was mental—a changed mind about my condition. I determined to do what I could do and leave the rest to God. Feelings always follow actions, and actions follow a change of mind.

Enlarge Your Vocabulary

Another way to challenge yourself in the mental area is to learn a new word each week to increase your vocabulary. At our group of Christian Life Communicators (a sort of Christian version of Toastmasters speaking group), we learn a new word each week. The person in charge of the meeting selects a word that very few of us know, then we use that new word whenever we speak at the meeting. The challenge is to work the word into natural conversation. Anyone can do this activity. Just take new words into your vocabulary each week, then use those new words in daily conversation. Some of us are so saturated in our regular word choice that we rarely say anything exciting. This exercise will help stretch your mental powers.

Discovering Balance

Read Regularly

Begin to read on a regular basis and it will increase your mental capacity. I tend to be an all-or-nothing sort of person. If I can't sit down and read an entire book, then I won't pick it up and read part of it. Yet if you read for only twenty minutes every day, after a year you would have read twenty two-hundred-page books. I find that volume of reading remarkable. Each of us can take a chunk of time and read for twenty minutes. A regular reading program would improve the mental aspects of our life.

If you are a poor reader or you don't retain what you read, consider this alternative: begin listening to Scripture memory tapes. Integrity Music produces a series of tapes with Scriptures on different themes set to music. One of these Scripture memory tapes is on anxiety. I listened to this tape for several weeks and not only memorized all fifteen Bible verses in a natural and painless fashion, but if I wake up during the night, I find the words to these verses playing through my mind. The Lord takes the words of Scripture that I put into my mind and reminds me of those verses—even in the middle of the night. You too can be mentally stimulated as you saturate yourself in God's Word by listening to tapes. Many wonderful books are also available on audio tape, including this one.

In First Place, we sometimes stress the mental area less than the other three areas. Mental growth, however, can have a profound influence on how successfully we handle the complexities of life. Some say "the battle is won or lost in the mind." When we give Christ Jesus first place in our minds, He can do anything with our lives.

PHYSICAL

"So whether you eat or drink or whatever you do, do it all for the glory of God" (1 Cor. 10:31).

The second area of our lives that needs to be in balance is the physical. There are four components of balance in this area: proper nutrition, exercise, rest, and stress management. Within First Place, we primarily focus on proper nutrition and exercise. The body is a wonderful creation that wants to heal itself. If people receive proper nutrition and exercise, most will find more energy than they have had in years. Regular exercise not only helps you sleep better; it is also a great stress reliever.

Years ago, everyone raised their own meat, fruits, and vegetables. The food was nutritious and people had to exert physical energy to get it from the seed stage to the table. In First Place, we ask our members to eat food as close to its natural state as possible. By natural state, we mean foods that are fresh, whole, and pure. We try to avoid processed foods because they are loaded with preservatives and sodium.

The primary physical motivation behind the First Place program is to develop and maintain a healthy body that can serve God as long as possible. The quantity of our life doesn't mean much when there is no quality, so our primary interest is not just getting thinner. Many thin people have high body fat, making them a walking time bomb for a variety of diseases. It is wonderful to be thin if it is accompanied by low body fat and lots of lean mass.

Many people start the First Place program to lose weight, but many others begin because of a health problem such as heart disease, high blood pressure, or diabetes. Numerous young couples begin so their children will eat nutritiously; they realize their children are simply following their poor example. Through First Place, a participant is educated about nutrition so it becomes obvious that he or she needs to make a lifestyle change. Our primary physical difficulty is not losing weight but gaining weight. Anyone can lose weight, but most of the time we regain it before we have had those new clothes cleaned three times.

Through the First Place program, you will not find quick weight loss. Most people who lose weight quickly soon return to their old way of eating and gain back the weight. Through a lifestyle change, participants achieve balance in the physical area of life. In any weight loss program, most people join thinking, *When can I stop doing this and eat what I used to eat?* Unless our lifestyle changes, we are doomed to the same patterns of failure. When you give Christ first place in your life,

Discovering Balance

He can bring about true change. As you admit to the Lord that you are powerless to change yourself, God steps in and begins to change you. Although many people experience dramatic physical changes (as you've already read about in earlier chapters of this book), in the long run, most of the participants in First Place say that the most important changes are in the spiritual aspects of their life.

We want these physical changes because we know that "man looks at the outward appearance, but the LORD looks at the heart." (1 Sam. 16:7b). As we look inside ourselves with God's perspective, we see our own misery. If we are overweight, we also know that anyone else we meet sees a body where God obviously does not have full control. Every sin is equal in God's sight, but the sin of gluttony is worn like a walking advertisement.

As you learn to eat right with a low fat diet that is very low in sugar, you must also exercise. If you don't participate in these two physical acts, then you will pay the price. Before I began an exercise program, I used to come home from work and lay on the sofa for an hour before I could even think about making dinner.

One woman in my First Place class had a brother suddenly drop dead from a heart attack at age forty-eight. Many of you reading this book probably discount this experience for yourselves saying, "It will never happen." Or if it does, then you will have angioplasty or heart bypass surgery. Unfortunately most people's ideas about heart attacks aren't based on reality. The most common symptom of a heart attack is sudden death. This man who suddenly died of a heart attack was a walking time bomb: he was a chain smoker who didn't eat right or exercise. Each of us has the opportunity to change our life and begin an exercise program, but we have to do it for the right motivation. Our primary motivation should not be for more energy or to avoid a heart attack but to please God with our bodies.

In my life, balance in the physical area is the hardest to achieve and maintain. Everyone has a lifetime of habits, which compose who we are as people. When we face times of stress, loneliness, boredom, anger, or even joy and celebration, we automatically revert to our old habits. Only God can retrain our mind and emotions, and thus retrain our bodies.

My solution for balance in the physical area is to continually make little changes and to have a mental determination not to return to the old way. For instance, about six years ago, I quit eating bacon, and now I am no longer tempted to eat bacon. In my life, the turning point for bacon consumption came one day when my husband said, "You know we probably shouldn't eat anything that will keep in the refrigerator for months."

Another part of the physical area that has been difficult for me is getting the milk that my body needs. I have never enjoyed drinking milk, so I struggled to get this nutrition for a long time. I've discovered that I like yogurt, and I also enjoy milk shakes made with frozen fruit. So for my milk consumption, I keep yogurt and fresh fruit readily available in my home.

Through the First Place program, you are never forced to eat foods that you hate. Every exchange list or serving list contains foods that you do like and you can select these foods. Since 1981, I have been living the First Place program and the changes to my eating habits have been gradual. This program will never make a real difference in your life until you transfer head knowledge to the heart. We each have enough head knowledge to eat healthy foods, but only time will change our feelings about these foods. From my perspective, First Place is a lifelong program that through the passage of time gives balance in every area of life. We must be patient and not quit before we achieve this balance. Our heavenly Father is extremely patient and merciful with us. Therefore shouldn't we be patient and merciful with ourselves? All true change takes time, yet time is what we resist so vigorously.

Our society wants instant everything. It will take time for God to teach us everything about a balanced life. True success is in the process—not the program. When we give Christ control of our physical bodies, we must ultimately surrender our fleshly desires. Our bodies naturally want their own way. Paul said it best in 1 Corinthians 9:26–27: "Therefore I do not run like a man running aimlessly; I do not fight like a man beating

Discovering Balance

the air. No, I beat my body and make it my slave so that after I have preached to others, I myself will not be disqualified for the prize."

SPIRITUAL

"But seek first his kingdom and his righteousness, and all these things will be given to you as well" (Matt. 6:33).

These words from Jesus are the foundational words for the First Place program. The spiritual aspect of the program is the third crucial area. It is only when we give Christ first place in every area of our lives that He can reveal His plans for us and make us into His image. Maybe you are saying to yourself, "Well when it comes to my life, God has His work cut out for Him." Trust me, no job is too big for God. Your responsibility is to release your own will and give God control.

When I was twelve, Jesus Christ became my Savior, and I became a Christian. Regretfully it was thirty years later that Jesus became Lord of my life. There were multiple reasons why Jesus was not Lord, but the bottom line was that I wanted to retain control of my own life. While I retained complete control of my life, I tied God's hands. He was always in my life, helping me in my marriage and in raising our children, but He didn't have the freedom to do His complete work in my life until I released my control.

This spiritual issue of control remains a mystery to me, yet from the evidence in my life throughout the last thirteen years, I wish I had turned it over sooner. My favorite Scripture is Jeremiah 29:11: "'For I know the plans I have for you,' declares the Lord, 'plans to prosper you and not to harm you, plans to give you hope and a future.'"

I can almost guarantee that the spiritual changes from the First Place program will be the most meaningful in your life. From my years in First Place, I have heard many weight-loss testimonies. In each case, the person is quick to say that the weight loss is great, but the spiritual changes are greater. God knows that we are created to bring honor and glory to Him. Until we fulfill our destiny, we can never live a balanced life.

FIRST PLACE

In the First Place program, we achieve a spiritual balance by starting every day with reading our Bible. Also, each day we answer one Bible study question that only takes a few minutes to complete. Everyone who participates in First Place learns what it means to have a quiet time and pray each day. In the beginning, you may only spend a few minutes in prayer, but as your understanding increases about God's love for you and His desire to spend time with you, your prayer time becomes longer and more meaningful. The entire First Place program is designed to take bite-sized pieces of time every day. It does not require hours of your time. When you understand that the nine commitments are for your good, you will want to continue each commitment in order to experience the benefits and changes that lead to a lifetime of good health.

An improved emphasis on prayer is one of the spiritual aspects where my own life has changed. My prayer life was so bad that I attended every prayer seminar that came into the Houston area. I knew there had to be some secret to a deeper prayer life that I was missing, so I was determined to find it through learning about prayer. Whenever I tried to pray, my mind would wander and I would think about anything other than prayer—my work, what I would eat for lunch—anything except focused communication with my heavenly Father.

I had always resisted the discipline of writing my prayers. "It takes too long," I rationalized. "Besides I talk faster than I can write, so it's more efficient." Then in 1990, I began writing my prayers in a prayer journal, and these blank page prayer journal books are now a part of the First Place program. My prayer journal revolutionized my prayer life. When I prayed without writing the prayers, it was scatter-shot praying, like, "Lord, here comes Mary and she's got a bunch of problems. Help me know what to say." I never committed quality prayer time to the Lord.

When I write my prayers, I often don't know where to start, but I pick up my pen anyway and ask the Holy Spirit to help me pray. One morning I prayed for a friend of mine who led a group at Sagemont

Discovering Balance

Church. The Lord brought this friend into my mind and I prayed for her—without a particular reason.

When I got to work, I located her address and wrote her a brief card saying, "I prayed for you this morning." Before too long, the card came back and every blank space was covered with her writing. She told me about that particular day and how much she had needed and valued my prayers.

Jesus set the example of prayer for us. He taught His disciples to pray when He taught them the Lord's Prayer. Throughout Scripture we see that Jesus never relied on His own wisdom, but on the Father's wisdom, because Jesus knew that He was living in a body of flesh on this earth. Look at an example in the book of Mark. Jesus had had an extremely busy day. He had healed many people, and I am quite sure He had gone to bed tired. But the Scripture tells that "very early in the morning, while it was still dark, Jesus got up, left the house and went off to a solitary place, where he prayed" (Mark 1:35). We too must pray continually to have the power that we need to live this life.

In First Place, we learn to give God the first part of each day so that He can control our thoughts and actions for that day. During our quiet time, we learn to read our Bible. This is the time when God can speak to us through His Word. I have learned through the years that whatever I am thinking or whatever I am planning to do must be backed up by the Word of God. The Bible must become the guidebook for every decision we make. We must become so acquainted with God's Word that we know the right way to think and the right way to act.

I believe our greatest example of how to live spiritually is our Lord, Jesus Christ. If Jesus needed to learn Scripture, then we should follow His example. The Bible tells us in Luke 2:46 that Jesus at age twelve had a profound knowledge of the Scriptures so even the synagogue elders were amazed at His understanding. Jesus was the Son of God, but He was also as human as we are. He had to learn the Scripture like we have to learn it. Only after we know God's Word and understand it can it make an impact on our lives. By memorizing Scripture, we have ready ammunition when tempted or when we need to quote the Scriptures to help someone else. Just like the other areas of balance, this takes time. We must be patient and give God permission to change us, and He will.

EMOTIONAL

The final area to bring into balance is our emotions. Each of us longs to attain balance in our emotional life. A few fortunate people have found emotional balance because they come from stable, loving families. If you are reading this book and the last sentence rings true for you, then you should celebrate the blessings of God in your life. I believe Luke 12:48b speaks of these emotionally balanced people when it says, "From everyone who has been given much, much will be demanded; and from the one who has been entrusted with much, much more will be asked." It is rare to find anyone in our society who has emotional stability. Families are disintegrating at a rapid rate, and children are the victims of the breakup. A friend of mine, Dr. William Heston, says, "Not everybody came from dysfunctional homes, but everybody's home had some level of dysfunction. It's a matter of degrees."[1]

Many of us live totally out of our emotions. We eat because of our emotional state—if we are happy, we eat; if we are sad or depressed, then we eat. Food is used to celebrate important occasions and eating becomes tied to our emotions. Many obese men and women have suffered from some form of abuse—physical, mental, emotional, or sexual. At our First Place program at First Baptist Houston, we offer First Place support courses as well. Through these courses participants experience emotional healing. Only God can heal the emotional wounds of our past. Many of us have been taught that healing is instantaneous at the time of our salvation, so we should be able to forget about the emotional wounds from our past. This teaching is misleading because emotional healing is a process and not instantaneous. Our salvation is the *beginning* of the process to become whole people emotionally. God longs to heal us of our emotional pain, and we are

Discovering Balance

the only ones who can willingly give our pain to the Lord and permit our heavenly Father to deal with it. The act of surrender sounds simplistic and easy but it takes a long time. Many survivors of abuse, whether sexual, emotional, physical, or mental, use the illustration that the healing is like "God pulling back layer after layer as we can stand the pain." Our God is as gentle in the emotional area as He is in every one of the other areas of our life. The pace of our emotional healing will never be faster than we choose. Still, God can't begin the process until we surrender our emotions into His capable hands.

I wish I could tell you that I have the emotional area of my life totally under control—but it's not true. Like you, my emotions ebb and flow. One week several years ago, when I was particularly down in the dumps, these negative feelings grew until I thought, *I can't even go into work. I can't smile or say anything, so I should stay home and regroup.* About 9:30 A.M. my husband was about to leave for work, and I had predetermined not to answer my telephone for the rest of the day.

As Johnny was walking out the door, the phone rang and he said, "Do you want me to answer it?"

I said, "Yes, please." When he learned who was on the phone, he told me the name. I thought it was a friend of mine (someone else) so I took the phone, and Johnny walked out the door. On the phone was a woman who I had been lifting to the Lord in prayer for the last six months. I had asked God specifically to have her call me. I had told God, "I don't want to call her because You have all the power. If you want me to talk with her, then have her call me."

God has a great sense of humor because the woman called me on one of my lowest emotional days of the year. I had been boo-hooing and feeling sorry for myself about my awful day, then she called. I began to feel excited hearing her voice, and we talked for the next two hours. By the time I hung up the phone, my negative emotions had fled. God orchestrated that phone call, then He gave me the emotional strength to handle the situation.

The Bible exhorts us to be prepared to talk about the Lord in season and out of season (2 Tim. 4:2). Personally, I'd rather talk with people in season than out of season. It used to be that almost every time I needed to give a speech, it came during my PMS time of the month. Everything in the day seemed black and horrible, yet in the midst of it all, God undertook for me and gave me strength. His power is manifested through our weaknesses. I could have blocked out those days from my schedule and refused to teach, but I didn't. God could not heal me of this emotional situation until I was willing to make a positive step toward emotional healing. When I finally gave up caffeine four years ago, PMS became an emotional illness of my past, praise God!

In First Place, we believe that to give emotionally wounded people only a weight-loss plan is like putting a band-aid on a cancerous lesion. Many people have never succeeded in weight loss because they haven't dealt with their emotional pain. In First Place, weight loss is not our primary goal. You may participate in the program for a long time before you find success in weight loss, but I promise that during that time God is working in other areas of your life. When we give the Lord first place in our life, He is the only one who knows what needs to transpire next. If you trust God with your emotions, then He will do the rest. Richard Chenevix Trench, in *Leaves of Gold*, said, "None but God can satisfy the longing of the immortal soul; as the heart was made for Him, He only can fill it."[2]

Within First Place, we constantly seek balance in life. We keep our four-sided balance symbol with each of the four aspects (mental, physical, spiritual, and emotional) as a constant reminder about balance.

In the next chapter we begin to examine the details of the nine commitments in First Place. These commitments are the heart of the program, and I'm anxious for you to begin. Let's continue the journey toward a Christ-centered life.

CHAPTER SEVEN

The First Five Commitments

Over the years, Carol J. White of Fort Walton Beach, Florida, tried almost every diet in existence. Her weight went up and down for years as she tried a fad diet that required fasting for one week, then only 1,000 calories the next, then fasting again. At one point, Carol took the drastic step of having her stomach stapled, which worked—for a while. She had given up on any attempts to keep weight off until a First Place group was started at her local church. The meeting was on the second floor and Carol's knees hurt with every step. She thought, *If I don't lose weight, I may not be able to walk in a few years—much less climb stairs.*

In August 1995, Carol, at age fifty-nine, began the First Place program. She weighed 267 pounds. The daily Bible study and Scripture reading along with morning prayer was a real inspiration for her. She says, "God gave me the strength and courage to face each day, and convicted me that my eating habits were sinful and that I needed to change. I went sugar free the first session, and I can tell you that only God could do that with me."

Since her first session, Carol has lost 92 pounds and led a couple of First Place groups. She emphasizes the importance of all aspects of the program: "My experience says you have to commit to all aspects if you are to succeed."

Commitment is an illusive quality in our world. It's almost impossible to get people to RSVP before an event. A more tragic example is evident in our families—at the first signs of relationship trouble, people drop their commitment to their spouse. The First Place program is built on nine commitments that when followed will draw you into a deeper relationship with Jesus Christ. In this chapter we will examine the first five commitments, which primarily relate to the aspects of spiritual health. In the next chapter, four more commitments will be explained, which are particularly related to the aspects of physical health.

These commitments are not listed in order of priority or importance. Each element is essential in order for First Place to transform your life into one of balance. None of the commitments is difficult, but each is important to achieve balance. Let's examine each commitment, then determine if God wants you to become a part of this program called First Place.

COMMITMENT 1: ATTENDANCE

"Though one may be overpowered, two can defend themselves. A cord of three strands is not quickly broken" (Eccles. 4:12).

Attendance at the First Place meeting is essential to success in the program. (We encourage you to seek a group in your area. See the resource page in the appendix for help in locating a group or starting one.) When we are not in class, we suffer, and the class suffers, because we need to meet together to gain mutual strength and encouragement. This commitment to attendance at the meeting means that we've made it a priority in our lives. We are committed not to let any other meetings or obligations take precedence over First Place. If for some reason we cannot attend, then we agree to call our leader or someone

The First Five Commitments

in the group. What would be a valid reason for not attending the meeting? Only the individual knows if it is a valid reason or not. (Someone once said that an excuse is a reason wrapped up in a lie.) A true reason for missing a meeting would be our own illness or the illness of a family member.

I once heard it said that 80 percent of life is showing up. This has proven to be true in my own life. I have to show up in every area of the First Place commitments. For example, in the area of exercise I can't remember a single morning when I woke up and said, "Oh, this is wonderful. I get to exercise today." On my own initiative—without any commitment—I would stay home, drink coffee, and leisurely read my newspaper. But one of the commitments of First Place is exercise, and I know it's important. Therefore I get up and show up for exercise. Some days, as I take my first steps, I say to myself, I'll only run a mile, but at least I'm doing something that 95 percent of the world doesn't do. I'm showing up. As I begin my morning jog, someone usually shows up at the track to jog with me. Invariably we begin talking and I end up running farther than originally expected. I know that if I don't show up early on the track, then it's a cinch I won't work in exercise later. And when I do, I'm glad I've kept this commitment.

The commitment to attendance is like exercise. You have to show up. If you refuse, your day will not be any better—in fact, it may be worse. This commitment to attend a meeting was written into the First Place program from the beginning. This small group of people becomes your support group, helping you to grow in Christ and change your lifestyle. During the first couple of weeks the group bonds; therefore, after this time new people must wait for a new session to start. This bonding is the glue that holds the group together. You will find that the individuals in your group form lasting friendships that extend far beyond the First Place class.

One of our groups at First Baptist Houston illustrates this deep bonding. After becoming a leader, one of our participants felt God's leading to emphasize a First Place group for women who weighed over two hundred pounds. Because she had been in that position, she knew

FIRST PLACE

the hopeless feelings these women often feel, and she wanted to reach out to them. At the next orientation session to help people learn about First Place, this leader put a little asterisk on the commitment forms handed in by women in this weight category. Then she called each one of them and asked if they would be interested in this type of group. Each of them expressed enthusiasm for the idea.

At the first meeting, she recalls, "I had never seen so much hopelessness in a room. These women had a long way to go and a lot of weight to lose. They were skeptical about their possibilities for success." The leader wondered if such a specialized group was the right decision. During that first meeting, the group began to get acquainted and bond with each other. As the women succeeded on the First Place program, pounds were lost and their spirits lifted. After a few weeks, one of the women asked, "After we weigh under two hundred pounds, does that mean we have to leave this group?"

The answer was no. The group stayed together. Their experience illustrates the deep level of friendship formed in a First Place group meeting.

Problems begin if we believe weight loss is the only reason to attend the meeting. If we have had a bad week and know we haven't lost any weight, or maybe even gained weight, there is a tendency to not want to show up for the meeting. We hope our subsequent week will be better, and we can show a weight loss at the next meeting. We are deluded if we fall into this type of thinking, because attendance at the meeting is the only way to have a better week. Through our attendance, we receive emotional support from other people. It reaffirms that with God's help, we can do the entire program. When we attend even during a bad week, we learn to be transparent enough to ask for prayer in our struggles. Our fellow members will pray for us, then call us during the next week to check on our progress. These phone calls and this encouragement from other people cannot happen unless we attend the meeting.

Also we must believe that God is still working in our lives—even when we don't lose weight. The Lord knows the plans He has for us, and they are not cookie-cutter plans where each of us has exactly the

The First Five Commitments

same experience. God works in each life in His own way because each one of us has been created differently. Our responsibility is to simply be available to God for His use.

From the beginning, this attendance commitment should be easy to accomplish. We must determine in our mind that we need each other and that is the critical reason that we've joined the group. Remember, success is in the process, not the program. If you don't quit, you will succeed.

What Happens During the Meeting?

The initial meeting is usually longer than the other meetings of the thirteen-week First Place session. Each subsequent meeting lasts one hour and fifteen minutes. During the first fifteen minutes, everyone weighs in, and their weight is recorded. People in the group say their memory verse for the week when they step on the scales. The assistant collects the Fact Sheets (commitment 7) and weighs in each member, leaving the leader free to chat with members while others are weighing in and saying their memory verse. All weighing in is strictly confidential and private.

Each meeting begins with prayer, then the leader guides the class in a few minutes of sharing. During this portion of the meeting, the participants ask questions or discuss any problems they are having with any aspect of First Place such as exercise, the Live-It plan, or their phone call. The leader might also share information from one of the First Place handouts. Next, the leader guides the group in discussion of the Bible study for that particular week. During the final portion of the meeting, the group shares prayer requests, and the meeting is closed in prayer. If time permits, the group stands in a circle, holds hands, and members may pray if they so desire. Members don't have to pray aloud unless they are comfortable praying in a group.

Why Should I Be Accountable?

Besides providing bonding, the First Place group holds each of us accountable for the weight-loss goals and other goals we set at the beginning of the thirteen-week session. Accountability is a concept that Jesus taught His disciples in Luke 17:3–4, saying, "So watch yourselves. If your brother sins, rebuke him, and if he repents, forgive him. If he sins against you seven times a day, and seven times comes back to you and says, 'I repent,' forgive him." By joining and attending a First Place group, you are accountable to your leader and the other members of your group. It's a responsibility that you should begin with a solid understanding. You are granting your leader permission to help you grow mentally, spiritually, physically, and emotionally.

Another reason for accountability is our presence in the body of Christ. The apostle Paul uses the illustration of a physical body in 1 Corinthians 12:12–26. In part, this passage says, "The body is a unit, though it is made up of many parts; and though all its parts are many, they form one body. So it is with Christ" (v. 12). Like our hand is physically connected to our body, in the same manner a First Place group is connected to each other.

When I lead a group, I am not a mean leader. In fact, some of the participants in my group have told me, "If you were a meaner leader, I'd do better in the program." I am not a diet cop, and I don't watch what people eat. Instead, my job is to encourage and motivate my group so they leave the meeting and return having lost weight. God will provide the daily strength, but the individual has to do the work of First Place. No one else can do it for them.

Some people refuse to be accountable to the group after they have joined. If that occurs, it means they may also have a problem with accountability to God. If they refuse to be accountable, then they don't weigh in or turn in a Fact Sheet or learn the memory verse. Maybe they rebel by not sticking with the food plan, saying, "I have to have my real Coke," or "I'm going to eat cake at the birthday party on Friday no matter what." If you are a leader and one of these individuals is in your group, don't take their rebellion personally. I have found that these people tend to refuse any sort of accountability.

Finally, accountability protects our freedom by limiting it. When you join a First Place class for thirteen weeks, you agree to limit yourself

The First Five Commitments

to the nine commitments of the program. When I discipline myself to these commitments, I am continually amazed at how well the program works! When we live and work within the confines of God's laws, we have real freedom that the world can't begin to offer.

Can I Do the First Place Program on My Own?

It's important to address this common question. We have had people who are homebound follow the program, and they have had great success. For medical reasons, these people simply could not attend a class. (Others may be unable to locate a group nearby and may choose to begin First Place on their own.) God honors their willingness to follow the commitments on their own, and they have succeeded in the program. Yet even in these situations they still needed to call a friend and discuss their struggles and/or progress.

I personally believe there is great power in the group. A group doesn't have to be large—maybe at first it is only two or three people. As we discussed before, the group brings accountability, and without the accountability of a weekly meeting, most of us would never truly get started. (First Place offers a leader's guide and video for those who would like to do the program with even two or three people and would like to have that accountability. Check the list of resources in Appendix I.) God has designed our lives for accountability. We know our bank expects us to have money in our account before we write a check. We understand that unless we come to work each day, we won't receive our paycheck for very long. If we understand this aspect of accountability, why is it difficult to understand accountability is the key for balance in every area of life? When you commit to attend a First Place meeting, you have taken the first step.

COMMITMENT 2: PRAYER

"If you remain in me and my words remain in you, ask whatever you wish, and it will be given you" (John 15:7).

FIRST PLACE

Personal Prayer Time

Your commitment to prayer is one of the most important commitments in the First Place program. When I began First Place, I didn't have much of a prayer life. I could do almost everything else but pray. When it came to talking on the phone for an hour, I didn't have a problem. At my work, I could concentrate for long periods of time. When I started to pray, however, I was easily distracted and began to think about my breakfast plans or what I would accomplish when I got to work. My mind wandered so much, that after a few days of trying, I gave up praying at the beginning of my day.

Instead, I prayed with shoot-up prayers. If I didn't spend time alone with God, then I shot up prayers during my day when I had a need. When I was first involved in First Place, I was not yet the national director. My work involved supervising the various secretaries in the Education Department of First Baptist Houston. One of the women I supervised was continually late to work. When she did arrive, she headed to the bathroom to put on her make-up. This girl and I did not get along, and early one morning as I was exercising, I shot up a prayer, "Lord, how can I get her fired?"

In a still, small voice the Lord said, "Carole, I love her as much as I love you."

I could not believe this response, "Lord, this can't be. She's obnoxious." Yet I began to pray that God would love her through me because I sure couldn't do it on my own. That day when I got to work, I knew where to find her—in the bathroom. I walked in and said, "I need to talk with you." She looked at me expectantly. I continued, "If I have ever done anything to hurt you, I want to ask for your forgiveness."

Tears welled up in her eyes, and she said, "Oh, Carole, I thought you hated me."

I told her honestly, "No, I want to help you be successful here." From that moment on, we became friends. Changing the way I prayed changed me and my attitude toward her. I learned that when I don't

The First Five Commitments

love someone, God can love that person through me until I begin to truly love him or her myself.

Shoot-up praying works in a pinch, but our heavenly Father wants a relationship with His children, and relationships take time. To have that intimate relationship, we must spend time daily in prayer with God. When you join the First Place program, determine what time of day is best for you to have a quiet time alone with God. Morning is my best time of the day. I wake up alert, and early in the day I can give my best to God. Your life may be different. Perhaps you have small children at home and no matter how much you try, you cannot get up in the morning before your children. If you identify with this situation, nap time might be your best time of day for a quiet time with God. If you work outside the home, maybe you can arrive to work early and have your quiet time at your desk. If you live alone, maybe you prefer to have your quiet time in the evening. Because of family obligations, evening is the most difficult time for most people. Whatever time you select, it needs to be when you can be alone. The quiet time for prayer loses its meaning with frequent interruptions.

Within the First Place program, we encourage the use of a prayer journal in your quiet time for several reasons. First, the journal keeps your mind from wandering. If my mind starts to wander, my pen stops. The prayer journal immediately brings my mind back to prayer so I can continue. A second reason for writing prayers is to provide a written record of what God is doing in your life. I love to go back through my journal and highlight where God has answered my prayers.

One morning during my time of prayer, I felt led to pray for one of our leaders in another church. When I got to work that morning, I sent her a note and told her that I had prayed for her. About a week later I received a note saying, "You will never know what it meant to me to know that you were praying for me that day. It was a witness to my spirit that the Holy Spirit impressed you to pray." Then in the letter, she told me about the various events in her life and how much turmoil filled every day. The Holy Spirit has the power to unite believers through the power of prayer. Through your regular use of a prayer journal, you can tap into that power source.

A third reason to write our prayers is to learn the natural progression for prayer. In First Place, we use the ACTS method of praying. If you write ACTS in an acrostic, it looks like this:

> A Adoration
> C Confession
> T Thanksgiving
> S Supplication

A—Adoration. When you begin your time of prayer, start by adoring God for His character and for everything He has done in your life. For your first attempt, you might find this awkward, but with a little practice you will find that adoration or praising God will elevate your mind to the right attitude for prayer. Sometimes I get a song book and read the words from a song to God. Other days, I sing a praise chorus to the Lord. The goal is to establish an attitude of worship in your quiet time.

C—Confession. After you have an attitude of praise, allow your heart to look inward. If you sit quietly, the Holy Spirit will bring into your mind anything that you need to confess to God. If you are a beginner in prayer, at first you might have to write down a long list of confessions and ask God to forgive each one. After you confess these areas to God, tear up the list as a physical symbol that God has forgiven each one. Now you are clean to go before Him in prayer. After this initial time of cleansing, you will find that sin doesn't accumulate if you go to the Father each day.

Confession and repentance go hand in hand. The Bible says in 1 John 1:9: "If we confess our sins, he is faithful and just and will forgive us our sins and purify us from all unrighteousness." When we sincerely confess our sin to God (which means we are sorry), then we ask God to forgive and to remove the sin from our life. If we confess the same sin each day, then we haven't repented and are simply telling God about our awareness of the sin. Confession is one of the

The First Five Commitments

hard areas in prayer. We like to make excuses for our sin. For example, we tell God and other people, "That's just the way I am." Often times, we justify our own sin, yet we are quick to point out the sins in others. Through true confession we come into a right relationship with God and move into thanksgiving and petition.

T—Thanksgiving. Philippians 4:6–7 says: "Do not be anxious about anything, but in everything, by prayer and petition, with thanksgiving, present your requests to God. And the peace of God, which transcends all understanding, will guard your hearts and your minds in Christ Jesus." When we begin to thank God for the many blessings of life, a peace fills our minds and hearts. We may think things look pretty bleak, but as we thank God for our health, our family, a home with electric lights and running water, then life comes into perspective. Henry Blackaby, the author of *Experiencing God*, wrote about the necessity of returning to our spiritual markers when we pray. These spiritual markers are times from our past when God did a mighty work in our life. When we thank God for our spiritual markers, it returns us to a place where our life is once again in clear focus. God wants our focus removed from ourselves and turned to Him. Our thanksgiving will accomplish this shift of focus.

S—Supplication. In our time of supplication, we ask God for anything that we need. For many of us, our entire prayer lives have centered on this portion of prayer. When prayers are limited to asking God for needs, then it becomes a grocery list, telling God what He needs to do for us.

A few years ago I discovered Isaiah 65:24, which says "Before they call I will answer; while they are still speaking I will hear." This Scripture has burned into my heart and soul; it has taught me that God knows my every need before I even ask. Yet even though God knows my needs in advance, I still need to ask. As another Scripture says: "If you then, though you are evil, know how to give good gifts to your children, how much more will your Father in heaven give good gifts to those who ask him!" (Matt. 7:11). Our heavenly Father is more loving than our finite minds can imagine. If you are a parent and your child makes a request, you will move heaven and earth to meet that request. There are many things that we would love to do, if our children would only ask. During the Christmas season I have seen parents go to ten different stores to locate something their child has requested. We love our children, and our heavenly Father loves us. He wants to give us the desires of our hearts if we will give Him first place in everything.

Corporate Prayer

A second facet of prayer in First Place is the prayer time at each First Place meeting. We believe in the importance of prayer, so we pray at the beginning and at the end of every meeting. Usually the time of prayer to conclude each meeting lasts about fifteen minutes. During this time, participants ask for prayer for themselves or for needs that affect their success in the program. We encourage people to limit prayer requests to personal needs. As you make yourself vulnerable enough to ask prayer for your specific needs, you will see the mighty power of prayer at work. One lady in my 6:15 A.M. class was having severe marital problems. Sometimes she barely got inside the door before she burst into tears. To attend the meeting, she had a long drive early in the morning. She would literally hold her tears in until she arrived at the meeting. Our group surrounded her and prayed with her so she could face the day. As a First Place group, we rallied around this hurting person.

Another element we emphasize with corporate prayer is that prayer requests stay inside the group. We ask each participant to never share a prayer request with anyone outside the group. As a result, the members of the group know their requests will remain confidential. From my experience, members honor this request and place the prayer needs into God's capable hands for His answer. When we have a safe place for our requests, we can voice the request and it ceases to have power over us. It has been said that we are only as sick as our secrets. God never intended for the Christian life to be private. Personal yes, but not private. Most of us have never been part of a group where we could be transparent and vulnerable, even, sometimes unfortunately at our own church. First Place groups are different because through joining the group, you have already admitted you have one problem in common. Either you need to lose some weight or you have admitted that you want a closer relationship with God. The group environment fosters honesty. Please don't misunderstand me; these groups are not a time for a pity party. The weekly meetings are extremely positive, but there is always time to stop and pray for a hurting member. Prayer is the underpinning for the body of Christ.

COMMITMENT 3: SCRIPTURE READING

"Your word is a lamp to my feet and a light for my path" (Psalm 119:105).

I am very grateful for Christian parents who took me to church and taught me God's Word. In church, we memorized the Bible and were taught to read and study God's Word for direction in life. This may not be your story.

You might join a First Place group and not own a Bible, or you might have to dust off an old one and take it to the meeting. Many leaders have purchased Bibles for group members because they did not own one. While on the surface our nation professes to be a Christian nation, many people grow up with no idea what the Bible says or how to apply it personally to their lives. While writing this book, I have been reminded of the enduring truth of God's Word in my life. God will bring a Scripture to my mind and insert it into the text. If I don't recall where it is located in the Bible, I can find the reference through my Bible concordance. This type of experience will be foreign to you if you have no working knowledge of the Bible. God cannot put something in your mind that is not already there.

The Bible will become a familiar companion that you open in times of trouble for consolation and help. As you read the Bible on a consistent and regular basis, you increase that personal relationship with your heavenly Father. Prayer is speaking to God, but Scripture reading is God speaking to us. It is probably more important that God speak to us than that we speak to God. After I finish my prayer time, I read my Bible because I am more in the frame of mind to listen to God.

The First Place member notebook includes a systematic Bible reading plan so you can read the entire Bible in a one-year period. You just look up the particular reading for each day. You can also use a *One Year Bible*, which is available in several different Bible translations. With the *One Year Bible*, the Scripture passages are divided each day into a selection from the Old Testament, the New Testament, Psalms, and Proverbs. I use the *One Year Bible* because it's easy to use and I read more using that system.

This commitment to read Scripture doesn't hinge on how much or how little you read each day. Instead, it is important to ask God to give you insight from the Bible that will help you in the activities of today. Sometimes after reading one chapter, or even a few verses, the Holy Spirit might direct you to stop on a particular verse. After you read that verse a few times, God may give you some insight into a current problem. Through that particular verse from His Word, God can speak to you. The Bible says, "All Scripture is God-breathed and is useful for teaching, rebuking, correcting and training in righteousness, so that the man of God may be thoroughly equipped for every good work" (2 Tim. 3:16).

Our goal in Scripture reading is to develop a systematic plan of reading. If you are unfamiliar with the Bible, you might begin with the Gospel of John. Read this Gospel several times until you understand what it says, then continue with another book of the Bible. There is no right or wrong way to read God's Word. The goal of this commitment is for participants to read their Bibles as a regular way of life. As you meet the commitment of Scripture reading, we hope God will give you a love for His Word that will last throughout your life.

COMMITMENT 4: MEMORY VERSE

"I have hidden your word in my heart that I might not sin against you" (Psalm 119:11).

The First Five Commitments

Each thirteen-week First Place session includes ten weeks of Bible study. Each week a memory verse is highlighted that relates to the study. During the week, participants commit to memorize this verse and to recite it when they weigh in on a scale at the weekly meeting. The memory verse commitment isn't a difficult one. If you participate in First Place for a full year, you will be able to memorize forty Bible verses. Scripture memory is important because these verses become valuable tools God can use when we face temptation or problems. He also uses these verses so we can help other people who are struggling and need our encouragement.

Once a preacher told his congregation, "Whenever you have a problem, you should ask God for a verse of Scripture to help you." The next Sunday a woman confronted the preacher saying, "Your advice about asking God for a Bible verse doesn't work for me." Then she went on to explain, "Three times last week I had a difficulty, so I asked God for a Scripture and nothing happened." The wise preacher smiled and said, "Of the three verses you have memorized, maybe none of them applied." For some of us, this story is all too true. Possibly the only verse you have memorized is John 3:16. Or maybe you have never memorized a single verse from the Bible. I have good news for you—it is never too late to start memorizing God's Word.

This summer I heard T. W. Hunt speak. He is the author of many books, including two of my favorites: *Disciple's Prayer Life* and *The Mind of Christ*. To my surprise, Dr. Hunt said that at the age of sixty-seven, he continues to memorize Scripture. He admitted, "Scripture memory has always been difficult for me, but I continue memorizing the Bible in spite of it." Then Dr. Hunt described memorizing entire chapters from the Bible. He memorizes these chapters also as separate verses so he can quote any verse in the chapter apart from the whole. As a child, I memorized whole chapters of the Bible, but I am not able to isolate a single verse in the chapter and say it. Dr. Hunt has accomplished quite a feat—especially for someone with difficulty memorizing Scripture. He also mentioned that he practices his memory work on his grandchildren. What a legacy Dr. Hunt is leaving his grandchildren! They will never forget the importance of Scripture memory in the life of their grandfather.

If you feel that you cannot possibly memorize the verse for the week, then write the verse five times each day and turn it in at your meeting. After writing the Bible verse, many people tell us they have memorized it. During your time in First Place, you should consider Scripture memorization as a gift to yourself.

Several years ago Martha Norsworthy, a First Place leader in Murray, Kentucky, told me how the Scripture memory commitment ministered to her during a desperate crisis in her life. Two days before Christmas, Martha's only daughter, Carol, and son-in-law, Bryan, were killed while driving the church van filled with Christmas presents to deliver to the families of their mission children. A woman who was drunk drove her car through an intersection and hit the couple. Their car burst into flames and they died in the collision.

At the time of the crash, Martha was leading a First Place group. When Martha arrived at the crash site, she knew there was no hope of survival. Immediately the Lord brought to her mind and heart that week's memory verse—Hebrews 12:1—which says: "Therefore, since we are surrounded by such a great cloud of witnesses, let us throw off everything that hinders and the sin that so easily entangles, and let us run with perseverance the race marked out for us." For Martha, this verse became like a huge billboard especially for her. Suddenly she understood that Carol and Bryan were in that great cloud of witnesses and that God had a race marked out for her. Martha's First Place group became her support group as she went through the grieving process. When this tragedy struck, Martha had already lost eighty pounds. During her time of mourning she went on maintenance without gaining back any of her weight. (Many of you understand the victory in this part of the story. As overeaters from emotional reasons, we surely would regain every lost pound in a tragedy of this magnitude without God's help.)

First Place members and leaders are not exempt from problems, but we know our strength comes only from the Lord. Christians do not

The First Five Commitments

grieve as the world grieves because we know the end-of-the-world story has already been written. If our loved ones know Christ, one day we will surely see them again in heaven. Martha said Carol and Bryan had been in First Place and that one of the precious items left behind was their prayer journals. On the pages of these journals, they wrote about the numerous changes God was making in their spiritual growth. Also these journals provided written reassurance for Martha that they were ready to meet God even if she wasn't ready to give them up.

As you begin First Place, you will be amazed at how God uses this commitment to memorize Scripture in your own life. Whatever you do for God is never wasted. God knows everything that you face today, and also the things you will face in the future. The Lord will use your obedience in Scripture memory to equip you for anything that lies ahead.

I have found some tips that make Scripture memorization easier. If you practice these tips, I believe Scripture memorization will become one of the joys of life.

1. Always state where the Scripture is found. Much of the Scripture that I memorized as a child lacks an address in my mind. Consequently, when a Scripture comes into my thoughts, I must locate it in a concordance. If you develop the habit of always quoting the book, chapter, and verse along with the Scripture, you will never have this predicament.
2. Scripture is hard to remember when it is just words without pictures. Anything that has a picture attached will stick in your memory. The other day, my granddaughter, Cara, reminded me of her struggle in second grade with her spelling. On Monday evenings she would come to our home, and we would make a game of learning her words. She recalled learning the word spaghetti because of the silly way I taught her to remember it. I told her to imagine a lady named Hetti with spaghetti on her head. Whenever she had to spell spaghetti, she would think of

spag-Hetti! In the same manner, you can do this to memorize verses from the Bible: just take the verse apart and insert pictures for words that are hard to remember.
3. After memorizing a verse, try to quote it when talking with someone. After you use the verse a few times in conversation, the verse will be more firmly planted in your mind. You need to repeatedly use a Bible verse to incorporate that verse into your life.
4. If you and your family memorize Scripture together, then when your children become teenagers, your job as a parent will be much easier. Psalm 119:11 says: "I have hidden your word in my heart that I might not sin against you." If you encourage your family to memorize God's Word, then this key information and insight will be in their minds and hearts to instruct them. Then when your children are troubled or have problems with peer pressure, you can remind them of a memorized Scripture verse. Better still, some of the teens that I know can quote Scripture to their parents when they are discouraged. God's Word will bond a family together in a magnificent way.

COMMITMENT 5: BIBLE STUDY

"Do your best to present yourself to God as one approved, a workman who does not need to be ashamed and who correctly handles the word of truth" (2 Tim. 2:15).

This commitment to Bible study is closely linked with Scripture reading. The distinction is that in addition to reading from the Bible, we study a specific area for the entire week. The commitment isn't overwhelming because within the First Place program, we answer one question each day. It only takes five or ten minutes. During the course of the week, we gain insight into God's Word for us. Then when the group comes together for our First Place meeting (or with your smaller accountability group of friends if you are not in a First Place meeting), we discuss the Bible study and what it meant to each of us

The First Five Commitments

that week. First Place has six different thirteen-week Bible studies and soon it will be increased to eight. With eight studies you could participate in the First Place program for two years without repeating a study.

I love to repeat the First Place Bible studies. When I repeat a study, I am at a different point in my spiritual journey from where I was the last time. It is incredible to me how the Bible, which was written thousands of years ago, is always relevant to my situation—today. The exact same verses will speak to me in a different way according to my current need. The Bible itself describes Scripture, saying: "The Word of God is living and active, sharper than any double-edged sword, it penetrates even to dividing soul and spirit, joints and marrow; it judges the thoughts and attitudes of the heart." (Hebrews 4:12).

Another means to dig deeper into Bible study is with some additional resources outside of the First Place study. The following resources will enhance your study time in God's Word. To spread out the expense, you may want to acquire these various books over a period of time.

Different Translations. Choose a Bible translation that speaks to you. Some of us grew up hearing the King James Version, and it is familiar. There are many excellent modern-day translations such as the New International Version, the New Century Version, or the New Living Translation. Spend a few minutes in a local Christian bookstore and try out some familiar passages in different versions; then select the one that speaks to your heart.

Parallel Bible. This Bible includes two to four translations. When we study God's Word, it is often useful to read several different translations because each one gives some different insight into the verse.

An Unabridged Concordance. This book contains an alphabetized listing of the words from the Bible. A concordance will help you to study different topics or words from the Bible.

A Bible Commentary. There are a wide variety of commentaries available, either in a single volume for the entire Bible or in multiple volumes. In a commentary, the author explains the Bible passage and some of the scholarly background. These commentaries will give you a broader understanding of the Bible passage.

A Bible Dictionary. This reference tool will give you insight into the cultural background of the Bible and help you understand definitions of difficult Bible terms like *atonement* and *sanctification*.

As an alternative to several of these resources, consider buying a good study Bible. Like the variety of translations, there are many different study Bibles available. Again, visit your local Christian bookstore and look through the various types. Talk with the salespeople to make an informed decision.

As you begin to dig deep and study God's Word, many new insights about God will jump from the pages into your mind and heart.

With these five commitments, we've covered many of the spiritual aspects of First Place. I hope you are beginning to see that these commitments are little bite-sized pieces that anyone can accomplish in a short amount of time. In particular, commitments two through five are the spiritual commitments—which every Christians should be doing already. From our experience at First Place, many Christians are not doing these commitments on a regular basis. Because they lack accountability in their lives, many days and months pass without any planned growth in the spiritual area. First Place offers an opportunity for gaining discipline in these spiritual areas of life, for those Christians in whom it may be lacking.

We've explained five of the nine commitments thus far. You've been faithful in our journey together through the First Place program. In the next chapter, we move into the physical part of our program and the food exchanges. Turn the page and let's continue our journey to a Christ-centered life.

CHAPTER EIGHT

The Final Four Commitments

For David Holmes, involvement with the First Place program was not a group experience. Over the years, David's weight had climbed until he weighed three hundred pounds. In February 1995, David was the minister of music at a church in Nesbit, Mississippi. He felt the need to lose weight, so one Saturday night David joined Weight Watchers and attended a meeting. The next day his wife, Melanie, saw an ad for First Place in a Baptist publication. The couple then located First Place materials in a bookstore. David began the program and committed himself to the nine different commitments. His accountability came from a couple of close friends and his wife, Melanie.

Like many people, David initially entered the plan for weight loss. His weight dropped to 192 pounds, but from his perspective the program exploded his spiritual life. "I had not consistently had a quiet time with the Lord before I started the First Place program," David says. Even while on the staff of a church, David had not consistently met alone with the Lord until he started the nine commitments.

After completing the first thirteen-week study on his own, David attracted some attention from others in his congregation.

FIRST PLACE

They asked him to lead a First Place group. He led a group through the first level of Bible studies while on his own, he completed the second level. For the next session, David led the group through the second study as he was completing the third one. David and his family are now in Decatur, Alabama, where David serves as the minister of music for his church. He was unsure when we talked if he would lead another First Place group in Alabama, but he was certain he would continue on the First Place program of Christ-centered health: "Initially I started for weight loss and that came, but the greatest benefit from the program was how my spiritual life was strengthened from First Place."

In collegiate basketball, every team competes to become one of the final four. In this chapter, we approach a different final four—the last four commitments in First Place. These four commitments predominately emphasize the physical aspects. In the pages that follow, we will consider each of these commitments in depth.

HABITS AND HOW TO CHANGE THEM

Because the majority of this chapter will focus on the physical aspects of First Place, it is valuable to spend a few moments looking at how to change our habits. Good and bad habit are formed through repetition, and eating habits are no exception. If you snack in front of the television, it's because you once did it for the first time. The next time you reached for a snack while watching TV, it reinforced the habit. You kept repeating the behavior until it became a part of you. Some other habits are: eating while reading, eating the minute you come in the house, eating when the kids come in from school, eating when you come in from a date, or eating while cooking dinner.

The Final Four Commitments

Also, we eat when certain moods and circumstances come into our life—even when we are not hungry. For example: anger, boredom, fatigue, happiness, loneliness, the kids are finally in bed, our spouse is out for the evening or out of town, nervousness, anxiety, our spouse brings home candy or ice cream—all of these may trigger an eating response. Our goal in First Place is not only to break these old habits but to form new ones through repetition. As you meet the commitments each day, you form good habits.

It is difficult to resist temptation; however, if you succeed in resisting the first time, then it becomes easier the next occasion. Before long, you have formed a good habit of resisting temptation. If you yield to temptation, you will find it easier to yield the next time.

Here are nine suggestions for new habits that you should develop. They will change your behavior if you consistently repeat them and they become a part of your life:

1. Eat three meals a day. Have two or three planned snacks daily.
2. Prolong your meals by: eating slowly, putting down your eating utensil between each bite and not picking it up again until you have swallowed the bite, hesitating between bites.
3. Choose a specific place in your home or office to eat all of your meals. This will become your "designated eating place" and should not be changed. Try not to eat at your desk at work. This would make you prone to eat all day long and not just at meal time.
4. Do not do anything except eat when you sit down for a meal. Do not read, watch TV, talk on the phone, work, etc. Make yourself aware of the food you are eating. Focus on the conversation and enjoy your meal.
5. Do not keep food in any room except the kitchen. Do not keep food such as cookies out on the counters. Do not store items in "see-through" containers.
6. Do not buy junk food. Neither your mate nor your children need it.

FIRST PLACE

7. If possible, serve individual plates from the stove and do not serve family style on the table. If this is not possible, put the serving dishes on the opposite end of the table.
8. Serve yourself on a smaller plate.
9. Develop a habit of leaving at least one bite of each item on your plate. If you can master this, it becomes easier to stop eating when you feel full. You will be used to leaving food on your plate.

Each of these nine suggestions relates to eating habits. Substitute another activity for your old eating habits. Some substitute suggestions include: taking a walk, take a long bath, call a friend, get out of the house, write a letter, read a book, do your Bible study, practice your memory verse, read your Bible, or begin a hobby such as cross-stitch, painting, floral arrangement, ceramics, woodworking, gardening, genealogical research, or sports.

COMMITMENT 6: LIVE-IT

"Do you not know that your body is a temple of the Holy Spirit, who is in you, whom you have received from God? You are not your own; you were bought at a price. Therefore honor God with your body" (1 Cor. 6:19–20).

"Live-It" is the First Place word for *diet*. The word *diet* is too morbid sounding for the Christian. The first three letters spell die. Life is meant for living, and the Christian's life—with Christ in first place—is meant to be lived abundantly. So let's "live-it," not "die-it."

Our "Live-It" plan involves a food exchange plan to help you develop good, balanced eating habits. We use the same terminology as the American Diabetic Association and call a portion of food an "exchange." The food plan is divided into six food groups:

1. Meat
2. Bread
3. Fruit

The Final Four Commitments

4. Vegetables
5. Milk
6. Fat

A well-balanced meal includes food from each of these groups. Many people believe that it doesn't really matter what they eat as long as they aren't fat. Yet I know many thin people who are in extremely poor health. In his book *Nutrition for God's Temple*, Dr. Dick Couey says that "sins against the body are costly. Our bodies deteriorate from heart disease, high blood pressure, diabetes, and cancer, which in many instances can be prevented by proper diet and exercise. You can neglect your body's physical needs, which often leads to poor health, or glorify God in your body, which often leads to good health. Your witness to the world and your well-being depend on the choices you make."

A key part of the Live-It plan is education. This section will help you understand some key factors about food consumption. First, there are approximately forty-five known nutrients our bodies need each day. These nutrients are grouped into six classes: water, carbohydrates, lipids, proteins, vitamins, and minerals. Unless we get these nutrients in the required amounts, our bodies cannot build strong healthy cells. Most of us don't know which nutrients are in which foods, so the exchange system has been developed as an easy way to choose good nutrition. Each food group includes a wide variety of food selections, and we know that each choice in a particular food group has basically the same nutritional make up.

Here are some basic recommendations for the Live-It plan:

- Whenever possible, eat fresh fruits and vegetables instead of canned or frozen.
- Use whole grain wheat products rather than white flour or refined products.
- Eliminate high-fat cheeses when possible.
- Bake and broil meats, and eat large quantities of fish and chicken.

FIRST PLACE

Within the food exchange, you select the number of calories you will need to eat each day. We recommend women eat no less than 1,200 calories and men eat no less than 1,500 calories. Many men and women have reported they never went below 1,500 calories for women and 1,800 calories for men, yet each week they lost weight until they reached their goal weight. In First Place, we don't want men or women to lose over one- and one-half to two pounds per week. The first one or two weeks you might lose faster because you will have a water loss. Afterwards, we know that if you lose more than two pounds per week, you are losing lean body mass. Lean body mass is your internal machine for energy and stamina. As a result, lean mass is not easily regained when lost. Within the First Place program, our goal is for people to lose only fat and not lean body mass.

Many people who begin the First Place program do not need to lose weight. These men and women experiment with the exchanges until they find the right number to maintain their weight. Most women can eat 1,800 to 2,000 calories per day and maintain their weight if they are exercising. The majority of men can eat 2,000 to 2,600 calories per day and maintain their weight if they are exercising. The goal of the program is for everyone to be eating nutritiously. Some will consume fewer calories until desirable weight is reached, but everyone will participate in the same food plan.

Because First Place is a balanced food plan, pregnant women and nursing mothers can stay on the plan by simply adding some exchanges. If you have a medical problem of any kind, we advise taking our food plan to your doctor. Then the doctor can advise you on how much food and which foods to eat. In First Place we never attempt to be anyone's doctor; however, it is important to note that medical professionals designed our food plan. If you have a health problem, it is likely the very same plan that your doctor will recommend.

What about Sugar on the Live-It Plan?

If people come into First Place and need to lose weight, we suggest giving up sugar until they reach their weight goal. We know that many

The Final Four Commitments

people are addicted to sugar and that when you are on a reduced calorie food plan, you don't need empty sugar calories. Each gram of sugar has four calories and absolutely no nutritional value. Honey has very little nutritional value also and is counted the same as sugar in First Place.

Sugar is not our enemy. If eaten in the right amounts, sugar is not a bad choice for occasional use. The problem is that we don't know what "right amounts" means. In 1900, Americans ate 6 pounds of sugar per year. The average is now over 140 pounds per year. That is 36 teaspoons per day. You say, "Someone is eating my sugar!"—maybe not. Sugar has been found in 94 percent of all packaged foods. Check your labels. (Four grams equals one teaspoon of sugar.) Here are some sample amounts of sugar:

Cola drink, 12 oz.	10 teaspoons
Ginger ale, 12 oz.	12 teaspoons
Fruit gelatin, ½ cup	4½ teaspoons
Cherry pie, 1 slice	10 teaspoons
Sherbet, ½ cup	9 teaspoons
Angel food cake, 4 oz	7 teaspoons
Chocolate cake (iced), 4 oz	10 teaspoons
Glazed donut	6 teaspoons

Unfortunately, because of the way food is processed, you can add sugar into your diet with little or no effort. It does take effort to monitor your sugar intake, and such monitoring is a key part of the Live-It plan. Bill Hybels in *Honest to God* uses a vivid example of our sugar consumption in the case of a junior high student:

> Let's say she starts her day with a "nutritious" breakfast of presweetened cereal. Mom is pleased she's eating cereal instead of a doughnut, but doesn't realize that one bowl contains 8½ teaspoons of sugar. That's a problem, especially when you add the 7 teaspoons in her white toast and jam,

and the 6 teaspoons in the sweetened cider she washes everything down with. It's only 7:30 A.M. and she's had 21½ teaspoons of sugar!

There's a midmorning break at school. Because Mom taught her well, she passes up the soda, but the chocolate milk she has instead adds 6½ teaspoons. At lunch time she enjoys a bowl of cream of chicken soup that has 4 teaspoons of sugar. A gelatin dessert adds another 4½, and a glass of presweetened lemonade contributes a whopping 8½ teaspoons.

On the way home, our growing young lady passes a convenience food store. Since her lunch was light, she stops in for a snack. No big deal. Just a package of frosted chocolate cupcakes and a soda—and 23½ more teaspoons of sugar!

That evening, Mom's too busy to cook, so she fixes a frozen beef dinner, complete with fries and catsup. That's another 5 teaspoons, and a small dish of ice cream adds 8 more. (At least she didn't serve cherry pie à la mode. One piece would have added an unbelievable 20 teaspoons of sugar.) Her total for the day: 81½ teaspoons of sugar—on a diet sadly representative of how many young people eat.[1]

If you look at the information, it's not too far from how many of us used to eat before we entered First Place!

Sugar eaten in the correct amount has not been found through research to be harmful. The phrase "eaten in correct amounts" is where Americans have a problem.

There are many names for sugar, and Americans are eating a lot more than they think. In First Place we ask you not to eat any product where sugar is in the first three ingredients. Ingredients are listed on labels by weight, so the ingredient that weighs the most is listed first and the other ingredients are listed in descending order by weight. Sugar is a little different on many labels because there are so many different names for sugar. The First Place member notebook includes a handout which lists every name for sugar. Through reading the labels and recognizing the terms, you can know how much sugar is in your food. Manufacturers have found that if they list the ingredients under the different names of the sugars, then they can have the actual sugar on down in the listing. You might see items such as corn sweeteners, fructose, sucrose, or sorbitol listed before sugar. These are just different names for sugar and sugar would probably be second on the ingredient list if they were all lumped together.

There are great benefits from removing sugar from your eating plan. Have you ever eaten an orange immediately after a piece of pecan pie? That orange will taste completely different when you have not eaten foods high in sugar. All fruits taste better and vegetables seem to have more flavor when sugar is eliminated.

America has over 14 million diabetics. Research says that sugar doesn't cause diabetes, but one of the factors leading to diabetes is obesity. How many Americans are obese because of the amounts of sugar they consume? Even though research has not proved conclusively that sugar is addictive, we have heard numerous stories from participants in First Place that eating even small amounts of sugar causes them to want more. For many, the hunger level is intensified. Also, sugar and fat tend to be binge foods for many people.

Each cell in your body and much of your total health is affected by your food choices. The goal in First Place is to provide your body (God's temple) with the nutrients needed each day to obtain the best health possible.

What about Sugar Substitutes?

In First Place, we have a key word when it comes to sugar substitutes—moderation. Most research is inconclusive about the long-term effects of sugar substitutes on our bodies. We recommend a total of twenty calories from the category called "free foods." Be aware of the total food products you use each day containing artificial sweeteners, including diet drinks. Also, consider the amounts of artificial sweetener you add to foods. Remember—moderation.

FIRST PLACE

Read Those Labels!

When it comes to food purchases, Americans are obsessed with the term *no fat*. The term gives us permission to buy cookies and cakes thinking there is no fat or calories. The truth is that most no-fat desserts have more sugar that their fat-loaded counterpart. If you read the labels, sometimes the fat-free product has more calories than the identical product that is not fat free.

Most of us don't take the time or energy to read labels, but in First Place we emphasize the importance of understanding exactly what you are eating each day. The most eye-catching nutrition-related information on food packages tends to come in claims right on the front or top of the label in relatively large letters. The following are among the most common and potentially misleading claims:

Percent fat-free. Consider a frankfurter that claims to be 80 percent fat free. Unfortunately, when a label says a product is 80 percent fat free, the words refer to the weight, not calories. The frankfurter is 80 percent fat free by weight but contains 130 calories and nearly 80 percent fat! This claim is true not only for frankfurters but throughout the supermarket. For example, one 97 percent fat-free yogurt is only 3 percent fat by weight but 24 percent fat by calories. To resolve this confusion, look past the "fat free" advertising to the nutrition label on the side or back. See how many grams of fat are in a serving, then decide if you want to include the product in your reduced-fat diet.

Light. For most products monitored by the USDA—meat, poultry, and products that contain significant portions of those items—light means the product is at least 25 percent lower than similar products in calories, fat, sodium, or breading (the label must state the exact nature of the reduction). When it comes to food regulated by the FDA, the term doesn't have to mean anything at all since that agency has yet to give the word a legal definition. Be warned about the false potential for this label.

No cholesterol. This is one of the most misleading terms in the supermarket and is found on everything from cooking oil to potato chips to peanut butter. None of those items ever had any cholesterol.

The Final Four Commitments

Cholesterol is found only in foods that come from animals and also in palm oil and coconut oil. These products do, however, contain relatively high amounts of fat, which has the potential to be even harder on the heart than cholesterol!

Natural. A natural product monitored by the USDA has no artificial flavors, colors, preservatives, or synthetic ingredients. It is minimally processed as well. What *natural* means on an FDA-regulated label is determined by the manufacturer.

No sugar added. This term is particularly confusing. First, it is different from sugarless or sugar-free. Both of those terms indicate a product does not contain any table sugar (sucrose) or any of several other sweeteners, such as honey. But the food may have sugar substitutes such as sorbitol, which contains as many calories as sugar yet does not affect blood sugar in the body the same way as sucrose. Sugar-free chewing gum and mints fall into this category. Items with no sugar added can have sucrose and other sugars as long as they are in the food naturally and have not been added to it.

The bottom line in First Place is that five grams of fat in any product except meat or meat substitute equals one fat exchange. Check the grams of fat, not the percent of fat. Remember that labels on products constantly change, with new and more detailed information being added to the label.

Another item not on the First Place plan is alcohol because it falls into the same category as sugar nutritionally. If you were going to count alcohol on the exchange plan, it would have to count as sugar or fat. Already you have learned that sugar has no nutritional value, and in First Place, fat has nine calories per gram; so alcohol is not a good choice for anyone wishing to lose weight.

What If We Stray from the Food Plan?

We realize that from time to time people eat foods not on the food plan. The difference in our philosophy and many other diet plans is that when we make a choice that is not the best for us, we are not off the program. This food is recorded on the back of our Fact Sheet, and at the next meal, we get right back on the program. Our old diet mentality told us that if we ate a candy bar or fattening dessert, then we had to skip the next meal. When we did this, we were doomed to failure. Since we felt like a failure, we usually ate everything else in sight before returning to our healthy food plan. In First Place, we know that now and then a bad choice doesn't make us a bad person. Food has no inherent value, good or bad. All food is good; but in many cases, our preparation of these foods is not good for us. In First Place, you will be able to eat the same foods your family has always enjoyed. You will just learn to prepare them in a different manner, using more spices and removing the fat. Also, we have many wonderful desserts in First Place that contain no sugar. Our members are never deprived of any food; they can choose any food to eat. The key is to learn proper serving sizes so you can be knowledgeable about your amount of food consumption. Many members tell us that they have served an entire First Place meal to guests and that their guests loved every bite. Often our mind-set of what is good food, and what is not, is totally unrealistic. We can educate our taste buds to prefer nutritious, low-fat foods. It takes only a little more work than it did in our previous manner of preparation.

Why We Need to Lower Our Fat

If you read through the food exchanges in the Live-It plan, you will notice First Place is a low-fat program. If we aren't really careful, most of us consume more fat than we need. Pastor and teacher Bill Hybels in *Honest to God* gives a vivid example of fat consumption.

> Jim started with breakfast—a three-egg, ham and cheese omelette—and heaped 7 teaspoons of fat on the plate. He added 6 more for two slices of buttered toast, and 1 more for a glass of milk. He didn't even suggest bacon or ham because they are 90 percent fat and ought to be outlawed!
> Then Jim piled on 5 more teaspoons for a midmorning doughnut, and wondered how many men would stop at just

one. Imagine what a glob of fat a long morning break could add! His lunch was chicken à la king—7 teaspoons of fat—and more bread and rolls, which added 3. He assumed the average working man would pass up an afternoon snack, but thought he would probably enjoy an all-American dinner: roast beef with mashed potatoes and gravy. For three ounces of meat, Jim loaded on 8 teaspoons, and for potatoes and gravy, another 5. Roll and butter, salad dressing, and cake with frosting each meant 3 more. A glass of milk added 1. The day's grand total was 50.[2]

One of the resources in the First Place catalog is a plastic model of a pound of fat. If you doubt this story about Jim, then you need to get one of these models and put it in a prominent place in your kitchen. It will be a constant reminder of the need to cut back on fat. (See Appendix I for ordering information.)

Water Is Important to the Live-It Commitment

Besides the Live-It food plan, we aim to drink at least eight glasses of water each day. If you have a 32-ounce insulated mug, you need to drink two of these each day. While it sounds incredible, water is quite possibly the single most important catalyst in losing weight and keeping it off. Most of us take it for granted, yet water may be the only true "magic potion" for permanent weight loss. Here are a few of the many reasons it is important to drink water for your weight loss.

- Water suppresses the appetite naturally and helps the body metabolize stored fat. Studies have shown that a decrease in water intake will cause fat deposits to increase, while an increase in water intake can actually reduce fat deposits. The reason this occurs is that the kidneys can't function properly without enough water. When they don't work to capacity, some of their load is dumped onto the liver. One of the liver's primary functions is to metabolize the stored fat into usable energy for the body. So if the liver has to do some of the kidneys' work, it can't operate at full throttle. As a result, it metabolizes less fat, more fat remains stored in the body, and weight loss stops.

- Drinking enough water is the best treatment for fluid retention. When the body gets less water, it perceives a threat to its survival and begins to retain every drop. Water is stored in extracellular spaces (outside the cells) and the storing is exhibited as swollen feet, legs, and hands. The best way to overcome water retention is to give your body what it needs—plenty of water; then the stored water will be released. If you have a constant problem with water retention, then excess salt may be to blame. Your body will tolerate sodium only in a certain concentration. The more salt you eat, the more water your system retains to dilute it. It's easy to get rid of unneeded salt: you drink more water. As water is forced through your kidneys, it takes away excess sodium.
- The overweight person needs more water than the thin person because larger people have greater metabolic loads. Since water is the key to fat metabolism, it is logical for the overweight person to need more water.
- How much water is enough? On the average, a person should drink eight 8-ounce glasses every day, which is about two quarts. However, the overweight person needs one additional glass for every twenty-five pounds of excess weight. Also the amount you drink should be increased if you exercise briskly or if the weather is hot and dry.
- Water preferably should be cold because cold water is absorbed into the system more quickly than warm water. Some evidence suggests drinking cold water can help burn calories.
- To use water most efficiently during weight loss, follow this schedule:
   Morning: one-third consumed over a 30-minute period
   Noon: one-third consumed over a 30-minute period
   Evening: one-third consumed between five and six o'clock

The Final Four Commitments

In an ideal situation, a person drinks a glass or two of water at a time. Space these drinks out over morning, noon, and evening.

- When the body gets the water it needs to function optimally, its fluids are perfectly balanced. If you stop drinking enough water, your body fluids will be thrown out of balance again, and you may experience fluid retention, unexplained weight gain, and loss of thirst.

As you begin eating and drinking the First Place way, you will never want to return to your old habits. You are in for a treat, not a trial.

COMMITMENT 7: FACT SHEETS

"Commit to the Lord whatever you do, and your plans will succeed" (Prov. 16:3).

As a participant in First Place, every day you fill out a Fact Sheet. (See page 197–198 for an example of this form.) Essentially a Fact Sheet is a food diary. On it, you record not only what items you eat but also the amount. This record allows you to record your difficulties with food and your victories over food temptation. If you are completely honest on your Fact Sheet, it shows exactly which foods you lack and areas where you overeat. The Fact Sheet reveals what you are doing and what you are failing to do in all the nine commitment areas. Every good, sound weight-loss program has some method of keeping a record of your progress.

Fact Sheets Keep Us Honest

When I became a leader, I wasn't filling out my Fact Sheet each day. During the leaders' meetings on Wednesday nights, I tried to reconstruct my food consumption over the previous week. During one of these meetings, Dottie Brewer said, "It's kind of hard to reconstruct a whole week in five minutes, isn't it, Carole?"

FIRST PLACE

I got the point! Even today, sixteen years after starting First Place, I find it necessary to keep a Fact Sheet so I stay on the Live-It plan. If I don't keep a Fact Sheet, I have trouble sticking to the plan.

At your weekly group meeting, you turn in your Fact Sheet to your leader for evaluation. Then the Fact Sheet becomes a method of communication between you and your leader. Accountability is stressed in the program, not so your leader can judge or criticize you, but to encourage you to make good choices. One of our leaders refers to the Fact Sheet as her "best friend." This single form captures each one of the nine commitments as a helpful daily reminder. Consider your Fact Sheet as a good friend. (If you do not attend a First Place group, find someone to share your Fact Sheet with to keep yourself accountable.)

Accountability keeps us on track. When we write those sugary desserts on the back of our Fact Sheet, it keeps us from wanting to eat them. Anytime we eat something that is not on the program, we need to record it on the back of the Fact Sheet. In the past, you may have been on diet plans where if you ate a candy bar, you skipped lunch to stay within your calorie count for the day. In First Place, if you eat a candy bar or anything with sugar in it, you still record it on the back of the Fact Sheet. At your next meal, practice good nutrition and eat what you're supposed to eat. This habit sets your mind on doing the right thing. While you may have exceeded your calories for the day, that's not going to make a great difference if you don't routinely stray from the plan.

Fact Sheets Reveal Trends

We can hide so much from ourselves. For example, we may be eating larger amounts than needed. When we measure and weigh our food portions, the truth is revealed to us. John 8:32 tells us: "The truth will set you free." In this particular passage, John was not speaking about food. Nonetheless, the truth about what we eat, how much we eat, and why we eat can free us from our bondage to food.

Every day your body needs forty-five different nutrients. Twelve hundred calories is the minimum you can eat to get these nutrients. If you don't eat all of the foods on the exchange list, you're going to lack

The Final Four Commitments

some of the vitamins and minerals you need. Some of these nutrients the body does not store, so our daily food intake is vitally important to good health.

Avoid consistently putting zeros in any category. Sometimes a person's Fact Sheet will have twenty or thirty zeros, usually in the categories of milk and vegetables. Omitting areas turns First Place into another fad diet. You need a variety of foods on your Fact Sheet. The beauty of the exchange program is that you find food in each group on the exchange list that you like to eat. You are not obligated to eat food you dislike. Each of you should go through the exchange list with a highlighter pen and mark all the foods that you like to eat. The highlighted areas will reveal either the wide variety or the limited nature of your choices.

Next, try adding some of the foods you didn't highlight originally. Through the food exchange, many people have discovered new food choices. Asparagus, not a popular choice for everyone, was found to be high on one member's list when his wife prepared asparagus casserole. Other not-so-popular foods become edible choices for many of us as we learn that fruits, meats, grains, and vegetables have distinct tastes. Many of us have eaten foods covered with butter, cheese, or cream sauce for so long that we think everything should taste that way. You will enjoy the discovery of new tastes.

In addition to your food choices, you record the amount of water you drink. Your body needs at least 64 ounces of water every day. This amount is the equivalent of eight, 8-ounce glasses. If you are like many people who are not water drinkers, it is important to drink an adequate amount of water for good health. Some of us have used colas, fruit juice, tea, and other beverages to quench our thirst. Knowing the need for water and the effect of not having enough water can help us form the habit of drinking more water daily. When our body is used to consuming more ounces of water, we will have the desire for it.

Fact Sheets Reinforce Our Commitments

While the nutrition side of the Fact Sheet is important, the back is every bit as important. On the reverse side of the Fact Sheet you check when you've read your Scripture, had your prayer time, and made your weekly phone call. Also, this section asks about your type and length of exercise. This ongoing record reflects the extent to which you are keeping your commitments. These commitments are actually more important than which foods you eat. If you keep these commitments, eventually your food choices will fall into line. Then you can get stronger and become more committed to your Christ-centered health program.

Sometimes you may fail to start your Fact Sheet on the first day of the week, or you may skip a day or more— you may even skip a week! If you attend a group, and you don't fill out a Fact Sheet, we ask you to put your name on one and write a note to your leader explaining why you didn't fill it out that week. Your leader will want to know why you're not doing one of the commitments so she can pray for you. Whether you have a reason or an excuse, you need to have somebody pray with you about it so your next week will flow a little smoother. Sometimes there are definite reasons for not doing a Fact Sheet for the week. We are not looking for perfect people in First Place, just committed people.

Many people keep their Fact Sheets in their First Place notebook. Others find that keeping it in their purse or organizer—even posted on the refrigerator—is more convenient. The Fact Sheet is a valuable tool to help you, so you should use it in the best possible fashion.

After you reach your weight goal, you don't have to fill out a Fact Sheet. However, most of my leaders who are at their goal weight continue to fill out a Fact Sheet every week. They find that filling out a Fact Sheet is helpful in maintaining their goal. It guides us in making correct choices in all food groups. When you increase your calorie intake after you get to your goal, you will find the Fact Sheet to be a regular reminder of what led to your attaining your goal.

If this concept is new to you, then you are going to find that as you fill out your Fact Sheet, God will be providing the answers that you have sought for so long. Give the Lord permission to change your life through your commitment to fill out a Fact Sheet.

The Final Four Commitments

COMMITMENT 8: PHONE CALL

"A friend loves at all times" (Prov. 17:17a).

The eighth commitment in First Place is to make a phone call each week to one person in your group or an accountable friend if you are not in a group. The most important reason for the phone call commitment is to reach out to others. When we begin First Place, we've already admitted that we have one problem in common—we need to learn to eat properly. Also we need to exercise and probably acquire a consistent Bible study and prayer time. Since we are aware of this common bond, it becomes easier to reach out to other members in the group.

Why Should I Call?

From my years in the church, even in Sunday school, I've found that people find it difficult to talk with others about their problems. We need to move beyond the surface sort of communication that occurs in the hallway of a church.

As a member of a First Place group, we can be involved in each other's lives and take the time to care about another person. A simple phone call during the week can make an enormous difference in another person's routine. To this individual, it says, "This group is different. Within the confines of First Place, you can feel that someone cares enough to listen to your sorrows and joys. We want to be here for you."

Some people are afraid of making their first phone call; however, most have found this phone call commitment begins a new opportunity and ministry. It is important to keep this weekly phone call commitment. It amounts to one tiny step in love to reach out to others who need it.

Why Is Calling Hard for Me?

Most First Place participants find the phone call hard to do. Perhaps it is because we have been rejected and hurt many times in the past. We may have built walls around ourselves to keep people from ever hurting us again. I believe that God wants to begin emotional healing in each First Place participant.

Through my experience in First Place I have learned how to truly love other people. I have loved people to whom the world had already given a strong message that they would never amount to anything or be useful. Why should I bother with them? The general attitude of my generation has been: if people don't conform to what we tell them to do, then let's just forget about them. God tells us something quite different. He says He loves every individual as much as He loves you and me. Whatever the individuals have done or whatever sins they have committed doesn't matter.

God's Word teaches that there are no degrees of sin; one sin is not more horrible than another. God says all sin separates us from Him. That's why it's important that we not only confess our sin to Him, but we must reach out in love to those around us; then we can forgive those who have committed sin against us.

This process of reaching out in love to others takes time. You will not be able to do it overnight, but God will empower you to forgive those who have sinned against you. When we refuse to forgive someone, it's as if they were sitting in a chair strapped to our back and we carry them around all our lives. Our unforgiveness doesn't hurt the other person, but it hurts us tremendously.

The root problem here is love. Perhaps we've never felt truly loved or able to love others. When the teachers of the Law asked Jesus what is the greatest commandment, He said to them, "'Love the Lord your God with all your heart and with all your soul and with all your mind and with all your strength.' The second is this: 'Love your neighbor as yourself.' There is no commandment greater than these" (Mark 12:30-31). This command is repeated in three of the Gospels. If Jesus said that it was the greatest commandment, then He meant it.

Many of us have a problem accepting and showing love. Maybe as children we didn't receive enough love, or we didn't receive uncondi-

The Final Four Commitments

tional love from our parents, teachers, or significant people in our lives. As a result, loving ourselves, as well as God, may be difficult. We may find God's unconditional love, as described throughout Scripture, difficult to comprehend. Therefore, reaching out and loving others is difficult for us. Yet when we are filled with God's love, we are able to love others (see 1 John 4:21).

As we continue in the First Place program, we learn that God loves us just the way we are—warts and all. God doesn't leave us on our own, but as we turn our hearts and daily lives over to His capable hands, He is committed to conforming us to the image of His Son Jesus. If you find it difficult to reach out to others because of your hurt in the past, then you need to pray and ask God to show you one person in your group whom you can trust. Ask God to help you bond with one person that you can reach out to and who will love you back. God will honor your prayers and begin to teach you about His love. As He demonstrates His love through others, He's going to give you the courage to trust and love in return.

What Do I Say?

When you make that call to another First Place member, you already know you have a common interest. You can always begin the conversation with a typical First Place question, "How is your week going?" The person that you are calling may be experiencing a good week; then you can celebrate together. If not, don't feel the responsibility to fix his problems or make her week a success. Just listening and caring will mean a great deal to the other person. If you have a suggestion to share, do it in a manner that leaves the person free to accept it or not.

The phone call enables you to be aware of what's going on in someone else's life. This type of detailed conversation will not always happen on the first phone call, yet it occurs as you cultivate trust and friendship. Often we feel that our food temptations are greater than anyone else's. Or we may feel that our life experiences are such that no one would understand them since we are the only one who has been through it. Personal contact gives us awareness that other people have suffered like we have and struggle in the same areas. We discover that God has healed others, and wants to heal us too. As we are healed, we can become part of the process for healing in others.

Many people relate that they had a cookie or a piece of cake in their hand when someone called from their group. Some put the caller on hold while they disposed of the cookie. The Holy Spirit urged that call at the perfect time. Many times when you call, you'll hear, "I am so glad you called. You don't know what I'm going through right now." Or someone will call you when you are having a particularly difficult day.

Pray for the person before you call him or her. Don't neglect to pray together over the phone and praise God for working through both of you. A few years ago I learned to cultivate the habit of telephone prayer from a friend in Atlanta. Whenever I talk with her, she says, "Well, let's pray together." It has become such a blessing to me to pray over the phone with fellow Christians.

I hope that you will incorporate prayer into your phone call commitment. You can say, "Could we pray together before we hang up?" Ask God to bless that person and wrap His arms around them that day. Allow the other person to pray for you before you finish the phone call. I am always uplifted when I hear someone taking my name to God's throne of grace.

Prayer is now such an important part of my life that I never start a meeting without it. Nor do I conduct a counseling situation without praying together at the start and end of the session. God blesses our lives when we ask Him—and He wants His children to come to Him and ask Him! So don't neglect praying together with the people in your group. Then praise God after the meeting is over for the things He has accomplished during your time together.

How Am I Helped by Calling?

Through the ministry of First Place I believe God takes men and women who have suffered terribly but have started to heal and uses them to minister to others. Whether it was sexual abuse or a specific

The Final Four Commitments

health problem, God was present when they endured such pain, and He loves them very much. He not only wants to heal their pain, He also wants to use them to minister to others in the same area of suffering.

People begin to see God's love when they see His love manifested in another human being. God's love becomes real to me when someone who shouldn't care about me not only cares, but also loves me. Don't neglect your weekly phone call. Allow God to minister through and to you. It's as simple as picking up a phone.

COMMITMENT 9: EXERCISE

> Do you not know that in a race all the runners run, but only one gets the prize? Run in such a way as to get the prize. Everyone who competes in the games goes into strict training. They do it to get a crown that will not last; but we do it to get a crown that will last forever. Therefore I do not run like a man running aimlessly; I do not fight like a man beating the air. No, I beat my body and make it my slave so that after I have preached to others, I myself will not be disqualified for the prize (1 Cor. 9:24–27).

Exercise is the last of the nine commitments, and I believe one of the most significant. As I have said, these commitments are not ranked in order of importance because each one works in tandem to bring our lives into balance. Exercise is one of my personal favorites though, because it has changed my life in many different ways.

Not Everyone Loves Exercise

Many of you will love the exercise commitment, but many of you will exercise and never develop a love for it. Even if you don't love to exercise, I can assure you that you will love the way you feel after exercise. My Assistant, Pat Lewis, reached her weight goal without ever exercising. For over thirty years Pat and I have been friends, and we used to lead a noon First Place class together. She never liked exercise and never found the time for it. Several years ago, while attending another church, Pat joined my early morning First Place class. Often to tease me Pat would bring me articles that said exercise was bad for you, or that reported that someone had died while exercising. When Pat reached her goal, people in her church began to ask her to lead a First Place group. As a leader, she felt guilty about never exercising herself. As a result, Pat prayed that God would work out a way for her to begin exercising. A couple of years ago, Pat started working at the First Place headquarters and she drives about twenty-five miles from her home. Before long, Pat found that if she left at 7:00 A.M., her drive to work took over an hour. If she left at 6:00 A.M., she could zip in on the freeway, have time to exercise, shower, get dressed, and still arrive at work before 8:00 A.M. Last year when her daughter had her first child, Pat stayed with her for a week. Afterwards Pat reported that if she hadn't been exercising regularly, she would have never had the stamina to do her work during that occasion. Pat will tell you that she still doesn't love to exercise, but she loves the way it makes her feel.

There are a few things about exercise that I don't like myself. One is, I don't like to sweat. Sweating wouldn't be so bad except that my hair gets wet and I have to wash it every day after exercising. But exercise has become as daily as brushing my teeth and going to work. I can promise you that my day goes better when I go ahead and exercise than when I choose not to exercise. As I recall that 80 percent of life is showing up, I am motivated to exercise even when I can't muster any enthusiasm. Also, since only 5 percent of the population exercises on a regular basis, if you exercise three to five times a week, you join an elite group of people.

The First Place Exercise Commitment

The exercise commitment asks that you exercise three to five times a week aerobically. Aerobic exercise can be any exercise that elevates your heart rate to a training level and keeps it there for twenty minutes. We have included a chart in the Appendix G that will show

The Final Four Commitments

you how to take your heart rate during exercise so that you know if you are in the training range.

Exercise Aids

The following items are either necessary or helpful as you seek to establish a regular exercise program.

A Good Pair of Shoes. From my perspective you don't need to spend a lot of money to exercise. Although it is possible to spend as much on your exercise clothes and shoes as the rest of your wardrobe, all you really need are some loose fitting pants, a shirt, and a pair of comfortable shoes. I paid ten dollars for my first pair of running shoes, and they were some of my best shoes. Cost is not an indicator of whether a shoe is right for you. The critical factor is locating a shoe that fits: one that is not too wide, too short, or too long. Serious exercisers do not look like they stepped out of a fashion catalog; usually they look pretty grubby—but they are comfortable. Don't wait to start until you get everything perfect. Start with what you have, and God will bless you.

An Exercise Log. In 1985, I began using an exercise log when I started my running program. In October 1984, I began walking and after I could walk a mile in fifteen minutes, I began jogging. Running is never necessary to attain a good fitness level. I began running because it takes less time to run three miles than to walk them. We burn one hundred calories for every mile covered, whether we walk slow, walk fast, jog, or run. The goal is to work up to at least three miles per day. You can decide how fast you will cover those three miles. If you are just beginning your exercise program, you might think, *Three miles! I can barely walk to the car.* In the early days of your exercise commitment, if you can barely walk, then barely walk. Before long you will discover that your stamina improves and you can increase your distance to three miles.

The appendix includes "Guidelines for Cardiovascular Fitness" from Dr. Dick Couey's book, *Happiness Is Being a Physically Fit Christian*, plus Dr. Couey's formula for getting fit in a twelve-week period. Dr. Couey describes six different kinds of exercise listed and what you need to do each week to become cardiovascularly fit. Also the appendix includes twelve weeks of our First Place Exercise Log so you can record your progress.

I love my Exercise Log and I use it every day. The log lasts for a full year and gives a complete record of your fitness. If I miss a week, I just write across that page what was going on and why I couldn't exercise. At the end of the year, my goal is to never exercise less than I did the year before. That way I am always working to increase my fitness.

Christian Tapes. Every day when I exercise I use Christian walking and Scripture memory tapes. I find that when God's Word goes into my mind for an hour each morning, then the Lord can bring it out when I need it. Many times during the night when I wake up, I find myself reciting a verse of Scripture I learned while exercising, or singing one of the praise choruses. What we listen to most is what will be in our subconsciousness when we sleep. That may be a scary thought for some of us, with all the garbage we allow to invade our minds. Use your exercise time to praise God and memorize His Word.

Pulse Monitor. For my birthday, my husband, Johnny, gave me a pulse monitor which monitors my heart during exercise. It has a band that goes around the rib cage, and a watch that picks up the heart rate. With this pulse monitor, I don't have to stop and take my heart rate during exercise. I can glance at the watch and if it is too slow, I speed up; if it is too fast, I slow down. Pulse monitors can be purchased at any sporting goods store, but they are not essential for exercising. If you haven't been exercising, it won't take over five or ten minutes for you to reach your training heart rate. My pulse monitor helps me, however, because I have been exercising for many years, and I had grown lazy. I had a hunch I wasn't working hard enough and the monitor proved it! For me, the monitor has been as motivational as my Exercise Log was when I first began to exercise.

When to Work Out

My best time to exercise is in the morning because fewer people need me early in the morning. If you have young children, the morn-

The Final Four Commitments

ings might be your worst possible time to exercise. The other day I went to my son, John's, home. His wife, Lisa, had gone to his office building after dinner to work out, and John was watching their three little ones. Other times, Lisa works out early in the mornings before John goes to work. You will need to experiment and find the time of day that works best for you.

Many young parents use their children as an excuse not to exercise. Yet children love to go out and walk and ride bikes. There is no better family time than when the entire family exercises together. It thrills me to see moms and dads out exercising with their children. These children are learning a lifetime habit that will continue into adulthood.

Husbands and wives have also told me that they never had time to truly communicate with each other until they began exercising together.

Some singles have met their spouses while working out. Exercise is good for any age and at any time. The main thing is to pick a time when you can be faithful to exercise. If you can exercise regularly after work, then that is fine. Some studies have said that if we work out in the late afternoon, we are less hungry at dinnertime. Afternoons have never worked for me because there are too many things that come up unexpectedly to deter my efforts.

Dr. Couey has done studies with women who couldn't lose weight as a result of years of yo-yo dieting. Their metabolism was so low that they were stuck and couldn't seem to lose. Dr. Couey discovered that if these women broke their exercise into two or three times a day, it jump-started their metabolism. For instance, if you normally walk for one hour, then walk twenty minutes morning, noon, and night. This arrangement also works when you have lost weight and have hit a plateau.

Exercise Helps Our Organization

Exercise has many benefits beyond strengthening our hearts. One of my greatest benefits has been to become a more organized person. It

FIRST PLACE

defies explanation, but I can plan and organize when I exercise better than at any other time. I have never been an organized person and have always resisted being organized. After I started exercising, I began to receive some of my best ideas when working out. I could solve problems that seemed unsolvable. Scientists tell us that our endorphins kick in when we have exercised for about forty-five minutes. If this is true, then it makes sense that our mental cobwebs begin to clear and we start to think better after exercising. Some of us need this more than others!

Exercise Is Vital for Senior Adults

As we grow older, we think that we just don't feel well enough to exercise. But amazing things happen when senior adults start exercising. You have probably read stories of seniors who could barely walk and now they are running marathons and going mountain climbing. I don't personally know any of these people, but I do know countless senior adults whose lives have been changed—and even saved—by the exercise commitment. For example, my mother is eighty-four years old. Eight years ago at age seventy-six, she planned to go with our family on a beach vacation where we rented a beach house. All of my children and grandchildren were there, along with my sister, her children, and grandchildren. On July 4, the men were busy barbecuing while the women sat and visited. My mom began to feel bad and went inside to lie down. My mom never lies down unless she is extremely ill. Within an hour, her fever was very high. My brother-in-law, a dentist and the closest family member we had to a physician, checked Mom and said we needed to take her to the hospital. On Independence Day you can imagine how crowded we found the hospital emergency room. At 2:00 A.M. we finally got Mom into a room. Her temperature had soared to 106 degrees. She was diagnosed with streptococcal septicemia, a strep infection of the blood that usually kills people within twelve hours. This same infection killed Jim Henson, creator of the Muppets. Fortunately, we were at a teaching hospital and my mother received excellent care. She had eight to ten doctors around her day and night.

The Final Four Commitments

They were amazed that she was able to survive this raging infection that usually kills much younger people. Although hospitalized for ten days, she recovered. To my amazement, the doctors told Mom if she hadn't been a faithful walker, her heart wouldn't have been strong enough to withstand that type of infection. I use this story to stress that the time to get physically fit is now—not when you are suddenly ill. Then it is too late. When you are well is the time to get fit, even if you are not as well as you would like. If you think, *I'm not well enough to exercise*, you must start where you are right now. Begin by walking a short distance every day. God will begin to strengthen your body.

Now my mom is eighty-four years old and she is no longer able to walk for exercise because of arthritis in her back. She does water aerobics almost every morning with her friends at the condominium where she lives. She says as long as she continues to do the water aerobics, she can function. When she stops, her body gets so stiff that she can barely walk. Exercise is essential at any age.

I could continue touting the benefits of exercise for several more pages, but I'll stop here. Please make sure you turn to the Appendix G and see the extra resources, such as "Burning Calories Is Key to Exercise Benefits" and "Know Your Training Heart Rate." When you exercise on a regular basis, it will change your life. The only way to find out is to put on those shoes and walk out your front door!

We've completed the nine commitments and you have learned the basic program of First Place. In the next chapter, we'll discuss the additional programs within First Place such as Fitness Weeks, conferences, and additional training workshops. We continue our journey to a Christ-centered life.

CHAPTER NINE

Beyond the Basics

In the fall of 1996, Linda Kelley started attending a First Place group at First Church of Dover, Florida. Invited by her best friend, Sylvia Montefu, who had lost forty pounds, Linda wanted to lose weight and restore her energy and stamina. During the past year, Linda has lost seventeen pounds and continues toward her goal of losing about fifteen more. A Christian for many years, Linda celebrates her deeper walk with God through the First Place program.

At Linda's First Place small group meeting, her leader, Doris Haynie, always concluded sessions by saying, "OK ladies, I'll see less of you next week [because of the weight loss]."

As Linda says, "Yes, she saw less of me each week, but the Good Lord was seeing more of me each week as a result of the nine commitments in First Place."

During the summer of 1997, Linda and some other women from her church attended a First Place conference in Hollywood, Florida. To describe her experience at the

FIRST PLACE

conference, Linda says, "There was quality content and excellent information which was presented with humor, love, and conviction. I especially enjoyed Beth Moore as a role model and godly woman, along with Dr. Dick Couey, who, as a well-known physiologist from Baylor, could present medical information in layman's terms."

FIRST PLACE CONFERENCES

Once you've learned the basic program of First Place, you have learned the foundational elements. However, within First Place there is a much broader program than the initial groups. First Place conferences are held throughout the year in different locations, such as Nashville, New Orleans, Cincinnati, or Dallas. There are no prerequisites to attending a First Place conference. Some of the participants are leaders in First Place who want to receive additional training while others simply want to learn more about the program or a specific commitment. Leaders and their class members often attend these events to enrich their lives spiritually, emotionally, mentally, and physically. However, many people who attend our conferences have never been in First Place but want to learn about the program. Conference participants attend a wide selection of seminars that address spiritual and emotional growth, as well as seminars that teach members how to take care of their bodies. Examples of the wide selection of seminar topics include: "Helping Teens Give Christ First Place" or "Why Should Christians Exercise and Eat Correctly." Participants also enjoy a number of dynamic speakers such as Dr. Bobby Boyles from Oklahoma City, Oklahoma, or Dr. Dick Couey, professor of physiology from Baylor University in Waco, Texas, among others. The atmosphere at these conferences is electric and the fellowship with other Christians is a boost to your spiritual life. An added plus is the opportunity to eat three First Place meals each day and discover firsthand how wonderful these recipes can be. For specific dates and times, call our office at 1-800-727-5223.

GET FIT AT FITNESS WEEK

Besides the First Place conferences, several times a year First Place offers a Fitness Week program at Round Top, Texas. The times and speakers vary. The week-long conference includes inspirational messages, exercise time, praise and worship, and devotionals. These in-depth meetings give participants a chance to interact with various leaders of First Place and get their questions and concerns answered individually. More than anything else, these Fitness Weeks are a spiritual experience that boosts the life of the participant.

Recently Dianne Stone from Greensboro, North Carolina, attended a Fitness Week. She decided to attend the conference during a time when she felt a a great deal of stress from her life, job, son, and her First Place commitments. She was starting her second session of First Place and had lost 30 pounds. Now Dianne was beginning to feel burned out, so she planned to give her commitments a boost with a Fitness Week. A week before the conference, Dianne reinjured her knee and had surgery for a torn cartilage. She contemplated delaying her Fitness Week until another session but decided to press ahead.

During the first two days of the Fitness Week, Dianne suffered with a migraine headache. As she says, "I was not a happy camper, but by Sunday, things were looking up." One aspect of Fitness Week is to participate in a social fast with time alone with the Lord. Dianne says, "I was able to rekindle a love relationship with Christ." For Dianne, her time at Fitness Week was invaluable.

Another participant, Missy Deterling, also talked with me about her experience at Fitness Week. Like Dianne, Missy brought her own struggle to the week—an allergy infection which persisted the entire time so she coughed and felt sluggish. The highlight for Missy wasn't the excellent food, the exercise, or the terrific teaching—while she raved about each of these aspects. She says, "The reason to participate in Fitness Week is for a spiritual renewal, a camaraderie with like-minded Christians and plenty of free time to spend with the Lord. I came away with such a peace, a stronger commitment to my Lord and a renewed attitude that, as Paul says in Phillipians, 'I can do all things through Christ who strengthens me.'"

FIRST PLACE WORKSHOPS

If you want additional help learning the First Place program or want to know how to begin and lead a First Place group or program in your church or community, call our office to find out about a First Place Workshop in your area. We hold four of these at First Baptist Houston yearly; however, many more are now being offered around the country. The purpose of the workshop is a passion to see the ministry grow, and each one is hosted by a church with an active First Place program. Each workshop teaches such topics as the history of the program, the four-sided goals, the nine commitments, the mechanics of starting a program, what it takes to be a leader, meeting procedures, and the food plan. A First Place workshop may be a good way to learn more about First Place and give you the tools to begin a program where you live.

TRAINING FOR LEADERS

During our conferences and Fitness Weeks, we offer Workshop Leader Certification for First Place leaders who have led for two years. The training equips them to organize and teach other workshops in their geographical region. Leadership training includes six hours of classroom instruction and an evaluation of each trainee's presentation skills. After this training, a leader must plan and present a First Place workshop in his or her area, observed by a First Place representative. After a satisfactory evaluation, the leader is a certified Workshop Leader.

A MONTHLY NEWSLETTER RESOURCE

First Place also has a four-color monthly First Place newsletter that provides inspiration, motivational articles, fitness information, recipes, articles about nutrition and fitness, as well as conference, Fitness Week and Workshop information. Each month's issue features an inspiring testimony with before and after photos. The newsletter is available for a reasonable fee. To order, call: 1-800-727-5223.

MORE RESOURCES

First Place is continually expanding its program to include the entire family. Recently we launched a First Place program for youth. This youth program is designed for grades 7 to 12 and focuses on helping the participant learn about eating a well-balanced diet and keeping fit for a lifetime as well as putting Christ first place. The youth edition involves five commitments: attendance at a weekly meeting, daily quiet time, learning a memory verse, eating healthy using the Live-It program, and regular exercise. The resources also include two different member notebooks with Bible study, leader's guide, and a menu planner with portion cards

APART WE CAN DO NOTHING

The additional resources listed in this chapter help you continue First Place as a lifestyle instead of a short-term program. Our emphasis is to help you live in Christ abundantly. Jesus said in John 15:5, "I am the vine; you are the branches. If a man remains in me and I in him, he will bear much fruit; apart from me you can do nothing."

This is a key to my life: apart from God and Jesus Christ, I can do nothing. Throughout this book, I've given you many tools and guidelines, but apart from God's help for every step, you cannot succeed.

FIRST PLACE

With God's help, you can live in a manner that pleases Him. He may plan for you to lead a small First Place class. God knows your life and heart and whether you will participate or lead a class.

Class size is no indicator of the success of your efforts or of what God is doing. Some classes remain small, while others increase. We lovingly accept those God has given us and leave the results from First Place in God's capable hands. We do the work of God, but He brings the results.

During the last several years, I have become aware of God calling out to me, saying, "Don't just do something, stand there." You see, I want to do things for God in a proactive manner. The Lord appreciates my availability, yet He wants me to come to His throne of grace through prayer and continued trust in Him. As I do so, He guides my life day to day. He will do the same for you. You are not alone in First Place—except by choice. The First Place staff is readily available to help you with a wide variety of seminars and resources. We look forward to serving you in the days ahead.

In your future, do you have dreams? Let's explore our future plans in the final chapter along our journey to a Christ-centered health plan.

CHAPTER TEN

A Dream for Tomorrow

In May 1995 Paula V. Stacey of Monroeville, Alabama, made a decision. Her weight had increased until she wore a size 26 dress. As she says, "I was in terrible health and believed I was about to die of a heart problem." Paula's church was starting a First Place program and despite her apprehension, she attended the meeting. Her first time on the scales, Paula weighed 295 pounds.

She began the program and did everything by the book(s)—First Place and the Bible. She recalls, "After the first week, I stepped on the scales, and I hadn't lost an ounce. I went to pieces, but I kept on and began losing consistently." In approximately twenty-one months, Paula lost 140 pounds—she lost one hundred inches and now wears a size 10 or 12 dress. Besides her weight loss, Paula says, "I have grown so much spiritually by allowing God to empower me to control my eating and exercise habits. He has taught me discipline (the big D) in so many areas of my life. I am a changed person on the inside and outside."

From the beginning, Paula determined to complete all nine commitments. She says, "I believe if you are going to do something, give it your all." One of her favorite commitments is the memory verse. Initially she wondered how memorizing Bible verses could help her lose weight. She says, "Memorizing Bible verses gave me encouragement and the ability to stay focused on the enormous task that lay ahead. The Scripture taught me that I can't, but God can (Phil. 4:13)."

About thirteen years ago, I sat with a friend at a women's retreat at a church camp near Austin, Texas. I didn't know anything about the speaker, but many people have heard her since that time—Patsy Clairmont. She had recently started her speaking career and talked about carrying a little notebook she called her dream notebook. During this retreat, Patsy talked to the group about having dreams—something you had never thought about dreaming.

As I listened, I wondered what sort of dreams could fill my life. At that time, I had never spoken anywhere to any group, yet there was a tiny seed of a dream in my heart to do so. At the commitment time during the retreat, I prayed, "Lord, if you want to do something with this dream, I'll make this promise: if I'm ever asked to go anywhere to speak, if I can possibly say yes, I'll say yes." As soon as I returned to my office, the invitations began. Some of them were unusual. Once I spoke in a home where I sank so deep into the couch that I couldn't see my notes. Yet these small meetings allowed me to do something some call PIT—Putting In Time. Anybody with a dream has to go through the training and gain experience before the dream becomes a reality.

What are your dreams about your future? In the earlier chapters of this book, I detailed how you can lose weight and improve your spiritual life as you follow the nine commitments of First Place. You've learned a great deal about nutrition and read the personal stories of a few real people who have already made this same journey. These people found more than weight loss through First Place—their lifestyle was radically changed and their relationship with the eternal God was strengthened. My hopes and expectations are great for you. Is God

A Dream for Tomorrow

placing some dreams in your heart? Are you willing to go through the PIT, to undertake the hard work, training, and pain that is necessary for those dreams to become a reality?

Some of you reading these pages have already been through great pain because of your physical appearance. Your self-confidence is pretty low and your mental image of what is possible may be pretty small. Maybe your spiritual relationship is weak, and you've rarely prayed or read your Bible on a consistent basis. Or possibly you begin breathing hard when you think about walking up some stairs because the idea of exercise is frightening.

In this final chapter, I want you to consider the words that Paul wrote the church at Ephesus saying, "Now to him who is able to do immeasurably more than all we ask or imagine, according to his power that is at work within us" (Eph. 3:20). Another translation says that God "is able to do exceedingly abundantly above all we ask or think" (KJV). I have a vivid imagination and can dream up some amazing things—yet God in His great love is able to do more than I can think or imagine.

As you look to the future, I want you to consider three major points. First, you need to see beyond the obvious, then you need to pray beyond the possible, and finally you need to live beyond the temporary.

SEE BEYOND THE OBVIOUS

The Bible is filled with examples of ordinary people who were completely committed to God's leadership in their lives. Consider the life of Noah and the fact that Genesis 6:8-9 says, "Noah found grace in the eyes of the LORD. These are the generations of Noah: Noah was a just man and perfect in his generations, and Noah walked with God" (KJV). It took years of discipline for Noah to build the ark. His entire life focused on obeying God and building that huge boat—on dry land. If you are going to follow the nine commitments of First Place and change your lifestyle, it will involve adjustments and discipline. You will need to find some new disciplines that you may not possess right now—except in your dreams.

Before my involvement with First Place, I didn't have discipline in my life. I drifted from day to day, just seeing what fun thing I could be involved in next. Through First Place, I've been able to fulfill many of my dreams, but it took many daily adjustments and the pain of discipline. In 1987 when I started my role as First Place national director, I could not envision the growth of our organization. I could not envision myself committed to the disciplines of prayer and exercise. I had to see beyond the obvious.

Consider the great patriarch Moses. Face to face, Moses met with God so much that his countenance glowed! If you recall, Moses was a reluctant leader. When he was tending sheep in the Midian desert and went to investigate a burning bush, God spoke and called him to return to Egypt to free the Israelites. Moses had every excuse as to why he could not lead the people. Finally he said he couldn't speak well, so God permitted his brother Aaron to go with him. Later, however, when Moses was on the mountain receiving the Ten Commandments, Aaron allowed the creation of the golden calf.

Yet despite Moses' mistakes, God used him. One time I heard an older woman use the expression, "Just let him whup himself." God allows us to "whup" ourselves a lot if we are determined to act on our own energy and strength. If you want to lose weight through First Place and have tried other things on your own strength, maybe you've "whupped" yourself. You must let go and let God take over your life. He will use your life if you look beyond the obvious.

Or consider Jonah. He refused to listen to God and fled to Tarshish. God wanted Jonah's life and commitment, so the Lord created a huge storm, and the sailors threw Jonah overboard. A giant fish swallowed him and after three days, he was willing to go to Nineveh and preach repentance. After God released Jonah from the belly of the fish, he obeyed God and preached in Nineveh. The people in the city repented and turned to God. Then Jonah was mad because God answered his prayers, but not in the manner that Jonah wanted. The prophet had wanted God to zap Nineveh, and, instead, they repented. In our lives, our prayers are often not answered as we would like them to be. God isn't some puppet on a string that we manipulate to meet our whims and desires. He answers our prayers for change in His way, according to His will, and for His purpose in our lives. I pray that you will take your plans related to First Place and put them at the foot of the cross—where all ground is level—and ask God to help you see beyond the obvious.

PRAY BEYOND THE POSSIBLE

As you dream about your future and a healthy lifestyle, I hope you will also begin to pray beyond the possible. Prayer is our communication link to our heavenly Father. As the eternal God, He sees the beginning and the end of our month, our year, and our lives. My finite mind tries to figure out what God will do in a particular circumstance. But Isaiah 55:8-9 says, "'For my thoughts are not your thoughts, neither are your ways my ways,' declares the Lord. 'As the heavens are higher than the earth, so are my ways higher than your ways and my thoughts than your thoughts.'" From these verses, I know that God will not respond in the ways that I sometimes think He should respond. My job is to honor God with my prayers and listen as I read the Scriptures for His direction. The most wonderful part of this is that God's ways and thoughts work perfectly at the perfect time.

Through First Place, we have given you a solid program for a lifestyle transformation: physical, mental, emotional, and spiritual growth. I have no idea how God will work in your life, but I'm confident that He will work in all of those four areas if you will make the vow to persevere and not quit until you possess the victory. When we put God in first place, then He can help us pray beyond the possible. I hope you will place your complete trust in God as He helps you pray beyond what you can see for your future. If God had shown me what my future would become in First Place when I started in 1981, I would have balked and said, "It's too hard and there's no way I can live up to those standards and commitments." God in His patience leads us one step at a time. Possibly you have been through a tremendous struggle with your life and don't feel like you can pray beyond the possible. Romans 8:26–27 says that the Holy Spirit intercedes for us when we don't know how to pray. Ask the Holy Spirit to pray for you and take your petitions to our Heavenly Father. The days ahead will brim with excitement in your life. I'm personally excited for you as you take this step of faith and trust God to continue working in your life through His power and might.

LIVE BEYOND THE TEMPORARY

Finally, I hope you will live beyond the temporary. Our world is looking for the easy way out and the quick solution. In the introduction of this book, I mentioned how we use the microwave to get quick food. Many of us have tried the quick weight loss methods and the results have been temporary. Our weight has returned. The basis of First Place is a total lifestyle change. As you follow the nine commitments, then God transforms you to move beyond the temporary into a total change of lifestyle.

In January 1988, shortly after I became the national director for First Place, I read a passage in 1 Corinthians 9:24–27. It says,

> Do you know that in a race all the runners run, but only one gets the prize? Run in such a way as to get the prize. Everyone who competes in the games goes into strict training. They do it to get a crown that will not last; but we do it to get a crown that will last forever. Therefore I do not run like a man running aimlessly; I do not fight like a man beating the air. No, I beat my body and make it my slave so that after I have preached to others, I myself will not be disqualified for the prize.

We can't lead anyone else where we've not been. God has to bring us a few steps down the road, then we share with somebody how God

A Dream for Tomorrow

has taken us to this point and how He can take them too. As I read this passage about running the race called life, God drew my attention to the final verse of this section: "No, I beat my body and make it my slave so that after I have preached to others, I myself will not be disqualified for the prize." This final verse has become one of my life's verses. It helps me live beyond the temporary and follow the discipline of a Christ-centered lifestyle.

Many people tell me, "After the first of the year, I'm going on a diet." Why wait? Why not begin tomorrow? Oswald Chambers, in *My Utmost for His Highest*, explains that our battle is fought in our will. Most of us have stubborn wills that resist God's direction and plans for our lives. The Lord wants to transform our lives mentally, spiritually, physically, and emotionally. Still, many of us are lazy and living for a temporary solution.

Through the pages of this book, you've started the journey of a lifetime. It's not temporary and it begins with a single step. Let me congratulate you for not only taking that first step, but for all the steps to come. Above all, follow the key principle of First Place—put God in the first place of every aspect of your life.

APPENDIX A
Personal Testimonies

KAREN ARNETT
Evans, Georgia

When I was four years old, I went to live with my grandparents for a few months. When my parents came to get me they hardly recognized me. My grandmother had fed me very well.

Although I was a very active child I remained overweight. Looking back, I know I mostly overate from boredom. Diets wouldn't work because I used food to keep me busy, to comfort me, and to push down any anxiety that I had.

It wasn't until I found First Place that I came to realize that only God could truly help me. Only by committing all of my life to Him and disciplining myself could I overcome my eating problem. With the help and support of people who cared, I was able to commit myself wholeheartedly to God and follow the First Place program.

I started a weight loss program in December of 1994. I lost 68 pounds before starting First Place. But I still wasn't submitting to God completely. I still would overeat and I didn't exercise. I started First Place in May 1995. God has blessed me in all areas of my life since then. I have lost 245 pounds and $83\frac{1}{2}$ inches. I have gone from a size 56 to a 10–12. I have been able to maintain for three months now. At one time I had great difficulty just standing in the back of a room and talking. Now I am a First Place leader and I give my testimony at area churches. It is amazing what God has done in my life.

When I was overweight, I was not a testimony to who God was and the power He had in my life. I didn't use the power He had given me. But now God has used the weakest area of my life to exhibit His power.

I would like to remind each of you that each part of the First Place program is important. If we will keep all of our commit-

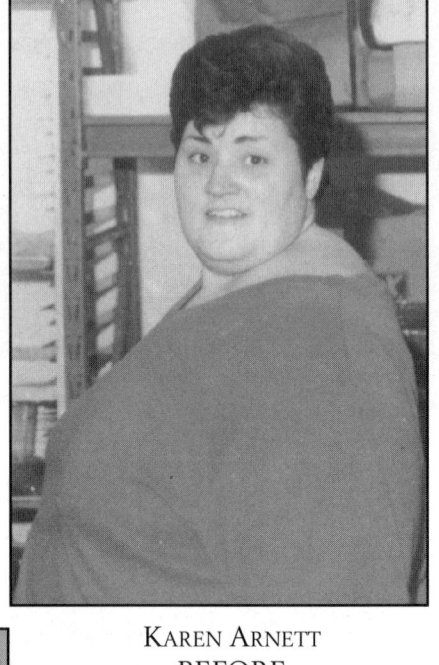

KAREN ARNETT
BEFORE

ments, First Place works. Each commitment builds on the others. Each commitment supports the others. Don't take your commitments lightly. You aren't committing to your leader, your spouse, or your friend; you are committing to God. God is faithful. He never breaks a promise. Each of the promises in His Word are commitments to us. He is calling us to faithfulness. When you make a commitment, you are making a promise to be faithful.

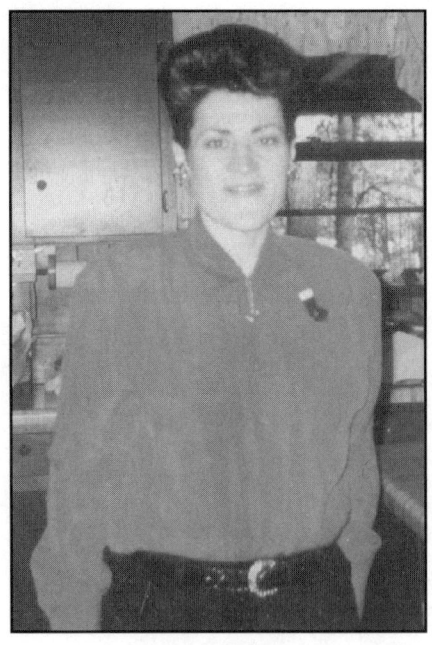

KAREN ARNETT
AFTER

Personal Testimonies

BETTY GRAYCE AVELSGAARD
North, South Carolina

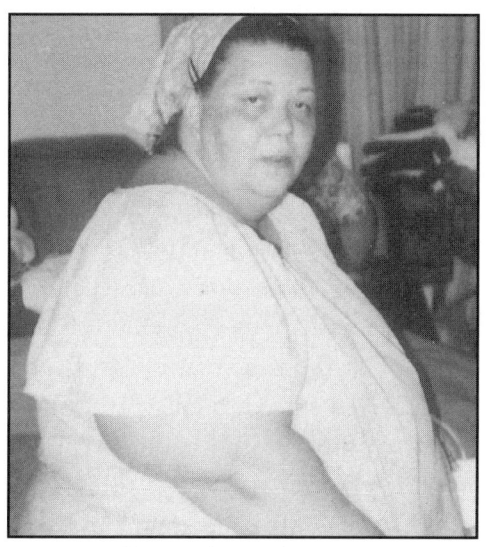

BETTY AVELSGAARD
BEFORE

Praise the Lord for First Place! You have saved my life. When our church started First Place in January 1995, I wanted to join, but my husband had been out of work for nearly a year, and it was out of the question. In September 1995, I was invited to the Victory Dinner/Introduction of First Place. I went knowing I still could not join. Praise the Lord, it was laid upon someone's heart for me to join and my membership was paid. Now the next problem—I couldn't weigh on their scale! It only went to 300. I was over 425! To make this a bit shorter, to date I have lost 159 pounds. I still have about 125 to go. I thank God every day that He loves me so much to put me among such loving people. Keep up the great work.

P.S.: My husband has lost 120 pounds because of my joining.

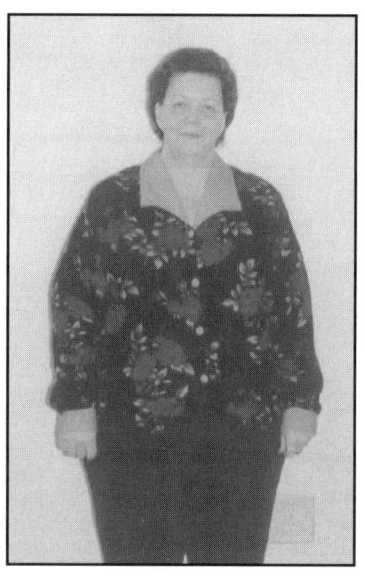

BETTY AVELSGAARD
AFTER

FIRST PLACE

CATHY DRESSLER
Newport News, Virginia

Throughout my life, many dates have stood out as dates that altered the course of my life. The date I became a Christian, the date I was married, the dates of the births of each of my three children, the date I was diagnosed with Parkinson's Disease. . . .

I had just celebrated my 35th birthday when I received the formal diagnosis of Parkinson's Disease, an incurable, degenerative, neurological condition. It was April 10, 1991, and I was devastated. Since the word Parkinson's had first been spoken in connection with what was "wrong with me," I had read all I could find about this relentless disease. The average onset of this disease at the time was 68. I was too young, it couldn't be true. But it was. I had a need to fall apart, totally and completely. I knew I needed to do this before I could begin the healing process and make plans as to the future. But all those who know my character and my strong faith wouldn't allow me to do what I so desperately needed, the re-occurring comment was, "if anyone can handle this, you can." Finally I did fall, broken in heart, broken in spirit, crying out to my Heavenly Father. In His infinite love and care, He wrapped His arms around me and lifted me up. I was reassured by His promise—I would be healed. Whether in this earthly life or in paradise with Him, I would be healed. And I will live much longer without this disease throughout eternity than I will ever have to

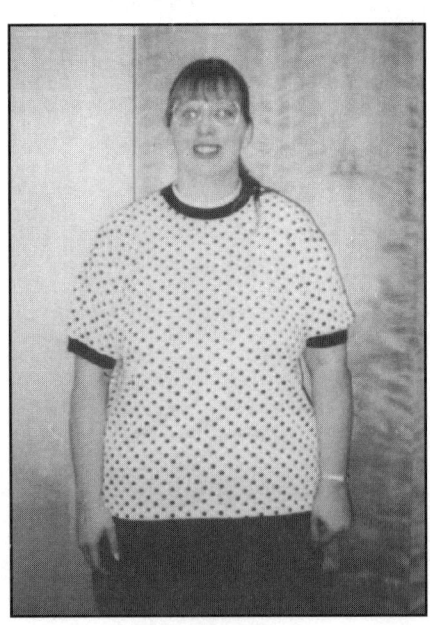

CATHY DRESSLER
BEFORE

Personal Testimonies

live with this disease. And as I live, my Father constantly reassures, "I am with you!" every moment, every day.

Soon, both sides of my body were affected by symptoms of Parkinson's—tremors, rigidity, overwhelming fatigue, and in my case, pain. I had to resign from my beloved job of teaching preschool. Through it all my faith stood strong. Walking became an effort as I concentrated on picking up one foot after the other. I began to drag my left foot so badly that I would often stumble, mostly catching myself, yet sometimes falling. But God would not let my spirit fall, His words, "I am with you!" were my constant companion.

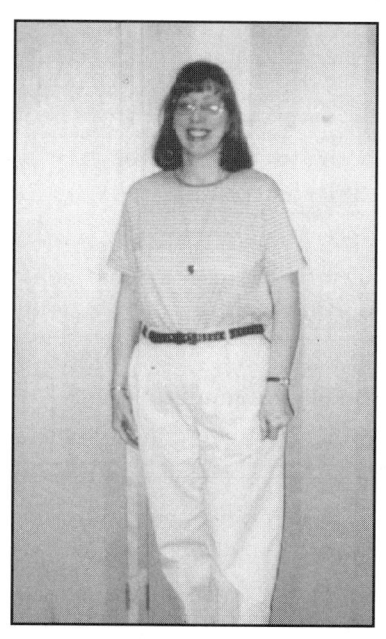

CATHY DRESSLER
AFTER

Orthopedic shoes and leg braces were ordered by one of my doctors at the National Institutes of Health. The brace literally lifted my foot from the ground as I walked and the shoes allowed room for the brace but also eased the pain caused by dystonia of my foot. Walking was not as hazardous but was still a tiring effort.

Already extremely overweight, I began to gain even more weight as inactivity became the largest part of my day. But I felt that my eating was at least one thing I could control. I could still eat what I wanted, when I wanted, even if I couldn't do the other things I enjoyed. Little did I realize I was not in control of my eating; it was in control of me.

But that all changed on the next momentous date in my life, June 11, 1996; the date of my first First Place meeting. The date I turned my vessel over to God. I had turned my life over to Him, my family, even my disease—everything—or so I thought. But I had not turned over the vessel for His Holy Spirit over to Him. What a truly beautiful revelation that was. God didn't see me as fat, as I saw myself and as the world saw me. He saw me as His precious child, and He was just waiting for me to release all of me to Him.

Everything changed! Food became what I needed as fuel for my body, not as an answer to every emotion, good or bad. I started slowly doing homebound exercises. But my determination to walk grew and grew. Not to just walk a block or two, but to walk a mile. That mile seemed to me as a marathon must seem to a runner, large and imposing. Just three weeks after I started First Place, I walked my first mile. It took 45 agonizing minutes, but I did it! With my First Place memory verses resounding in my soul, with the song "Onward Christian Soldiers" playing in my head—I had walked! Thank you, God! A few weeks later I walked one mile in 15 minutes! Praise God!

Then it happened. On a balmy summer evening as I walked with my husband, a verse from my First Place Bible reading that day was brought to mind. The verse from Proverbs 3:23 said, "When you walk, your steps will not be hampered; when you run, you will not stumble." Over and over the Holy Spirit spoke those words to me . . . "you will not stumble, you will not stumble." With each step my feet felt lighter, freer, and then, almost of their own volition, they picked up speed, my stride lengthened, and I was running! With the wind rushing through my hair, I ran for three blocks! My husband called out, "Go, girl!" and his words became intermingled with the sound of my Father saying, "I am with you!"

I have now lost 93 pounds and over 30 inches on the First Place program. I have a few more pounds to go, and I know I will be at goal. I'm now leading my second session and being blessed by each class member. I get so excited when someone asks how I lost the weight, just the opening I need to tell them what God has done for me through First Place. I praise God and give Him the glory for every pound lost, every inch gone, every step taken.

Oh, and those orthopedic shoes and the leg brace are now relegated to a dusty corner of my closet. And for this past Christmas, my wonderful husband gave me a new pair of shoes. What kind? Nike Air Windrunners, of course!

MARY ENGLE
Houston, Texas

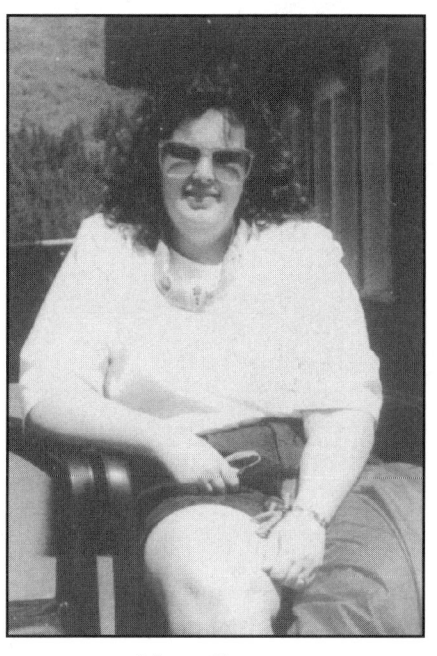

MARY ENGLE
BEFORE

Mother Teresa once said, "We are all pencils in the hand of God." Well, in January 1994, God picked up this old chewed-up, beaten-up, dull-pointed, #2 pencil and began writing a new chapter. I had been in recovery for childhood sexual and emotional abuse for about a year and a half. I had been back in church after a 10-year hiatus, consumed with sins too numerous to name. I was also in a very abusive marriage that left me feeling rejected and worthless. And I was feeling fat and ugly, ugly, ugly! But there I was sitting in a First Place group at Houston's First Baptist!

When I went into recovery, I thought when I lost all of my weight my recovery would be complete. Like many sexual abuse survivors, I had put on weight at the onset of abuse. Some people refer to the added weight as the "second layer" of skin because of the protection they believe it offers. For me, the additional weight confirmed my every thought. "I feel worthless. I look worthless. Therefore, I am worthless!" "I feel ugly. I look ugly. Therefore, I am ugly." Additionally, I put the weight on in hopes of discouraging any further advances.

But my God is a bigger God than any emotional, physical, or mental problem! I walked into First Place expecting to lose weight, and I did! So far I have lost 38 pounds. What is even more exciting for me is that I feel like I have lost about 100 emotional pounds! Through First Place, I have learned that our God is a God of second chances and third chances and fourth chances and fifth chances. I am also learning that balance is the key to my restoration towards wholeness. My emotional healing was a team effort between First Place and the professional Christian counseling I received. I have had so many of my First Place friends cheering me on during these past difficult years. One significant moment towards emotional healing came when my therapist encouraged me to stand in front of a mirror without any clothes on and look at myself. It was a gradual process for me. I was beginning to lose some weight and every once in a while I would stand in front of the mirror with my clothes on and say "O.K., this isn't so bad, I can do this!" The next time I looked at myself in the mirror I decided to really stretch, and I wore a towel draped around me. It was as if I was testing God to see if He would come flying through that mirror and laugh at my body. But He never did. I continued to seek guidance from my counselor and my friends at First Place. Combined with their loving encouragement and studying God's word in a way I never had before, I began to feel an incredible sense of unconditional love. The day came when I felt brave enough to look at myself in the mirror totally in the buff. I felt like Sally Fields when she exclaimed, "You like me! You really like me!" after she won the Academy award for the movie *Norma Rae*. Only I was exclaiming, "I like me! I really like me!" That is God working, for me to be at a place emotionally to say that.

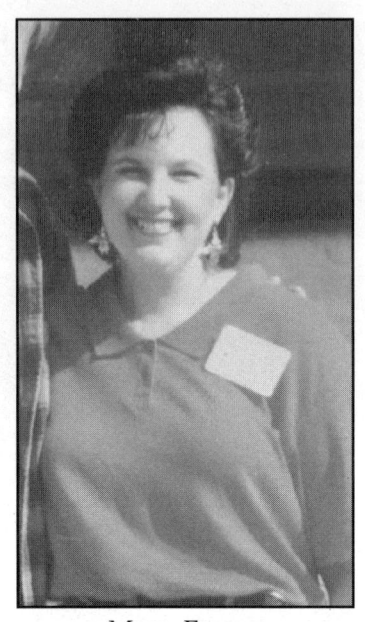

MARY ENGLE
AFTER

Amazingly enough, instead of that old pencil that God picked up getting duller, it got sharper and is continuing to get sharper! What does my chapter look like today in 1997? It looks promising. I am single again and stronger emotionally than ever. (My First Place friends

Personal Testimonies

have held my hand through a very difficult separation and divorce.) I am no longer a survivor of sexual abuse, but rather a victor. I am also using my experience in First Place and leading a specialty class for sexual abuse survivors. Thank you, God, thank you, First Place, and thank you me for loving me enough not to give up on this #2 pencil!

CAROLYN FERGUSON
Jonesboro, Arkansas

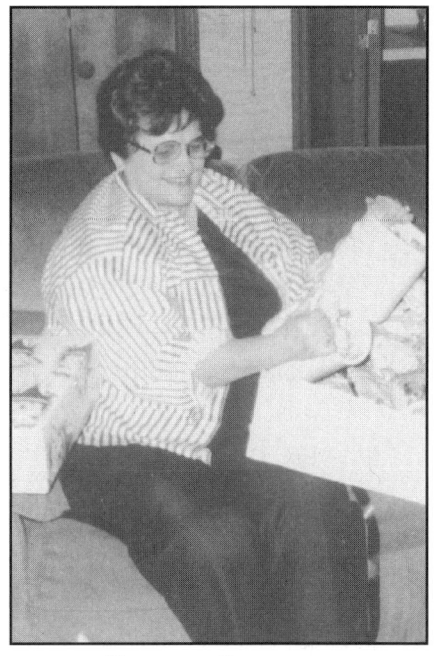

CAROLYN FERGUSON
BEFORE

I have been on the usual diets that most everyone else has, and like everyone else, I would lose a few pounds, then gain it all back. In February 1995, I began to have serious knee problems due to osteoarthritis. On the 18th of February, it was so bad I could not move it, bend it, and the swelling was bad. I weighed $234\frac{1}{2}$ pounds at the time. It took three adults to get me into the van to take me to the emergency room. I was so embarrassed. On the way to the hospital, I told my daughter I was going to lose this weight one way or another. I was so depressed. Of course, she supported me and offered to help in any way she could.

I had to have emergency arthroscopic knee surgery two days later. I had heard of First Place at our church but knew nothing about it. One of the ladies in my Sunday School class told me about the success she was having. I decided to give it a try. The next session was starting in April of that year.

FIRST PLACE

I was amazed at the results. For the first time in my life I was able to eat three meals a day, learn better Bible study habits, and had good Christian friends to support me to lose the weight. I really like the fact that they left it up to me how much I wanted to lose. There were no goals set for weight loss except the ones I set for myself. That was so much help to know that I only needed to work on the first ten or fifteen pounds. That really helped my attitude to get me started. Then the next session I could work on the next ten pounds, and so on.

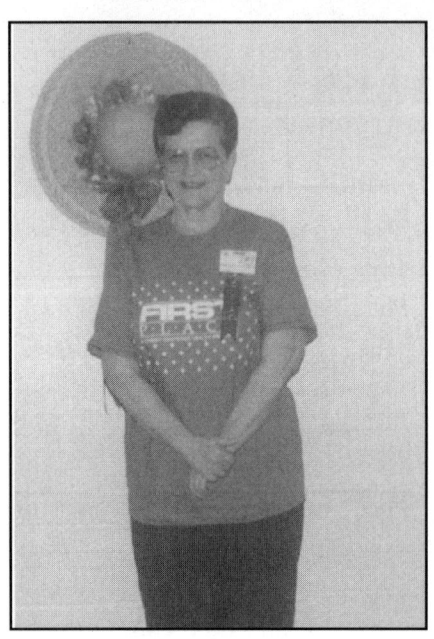

CAROLYN FERGUSON
AFTER

I joined in April 1995, mainly for the weight loss program, and by December I had lost over fifty pounds. In October 1995, I had to have total left knee replacement surgery. My knee was giving me so many problems, I was having trouble walking at all. Some days I did not. My doctor was so pleased I had lost the weight. He said that I would heal faster and better as a result and be back on my feet sooner than I would have if I had not lost the weight. He also told me that for every pound lost, it was three pounds of weight off my knee. Every time you step, you place three times your weight on your knees.

I did heal well. My daughter, Connie Coldwell, is a licensed physical therapist assistant, and she was my therapist. She encouraged me and worked with me until I was able to get around very well. I still have to do regular exercise to keep everything working properly. My grandsons, Nick and Andy, who were three and ten at the time, would

Personal Testimonies

hold my hands to help me handle the pain when I took the exercises. About the only thing I cannot do very well now is kneel.

I am so thankful for First Place, our leaders, and any of those responsible for bringing it to our church. I know without it I would still be too heavy, and my health would be a total disaster. It feels good to be able to sit and pull my knees up in front of me, to wear jeans again, and to buy off the regular size racks in the store instead of the plus sizes. Before, I could not do any of this.

For people who need to lose weight, there is nothing like First Place. There is very little food we have to do totally without. For almost everything we eat, there is a low-calorie, low-fat recipe. I just can't say enough about First Place—all good. You also make some really great friends who love you and support you when you need it. I have gotten to know people through First Place whom I would probably never have made friends with otherwise.

I decided to write my story in case it helps someone else who may have some of the problems I have. My family doctor and my orthopedic doctor have both kept track of my progress and both are very pleased. My family doctor was really pleased when I went in for a check up in January, and I had maintained the weight loss and even lost some more since my last check up with him a few months ago. I am looking forward to going to my school and family reunions which are being held this year. I have never wanted to go before.

Thank you all. You are all so special and I know God will reward you for all you are doing with First Place.

SHARON KING
Effingham, South Carolina

The Lord invited me to join Him in His work but first some changes were necessary.

For as long as I can remember, I struggled with a food and weight problem. Little did I know in January 1995 it was the beginning of the end of the struggle. In December 1994, after regaining a third of twenty recently lost pounds, I admitted defeat in the weight war. I decided I would not put myself through the mental and emotional torture of another diet—even if it meant weighing over 200 pounds. Two to three weeks later, a poster in my Sunday school class advertised First Place, a new program in discipleship training. As I read and re-read the information, I know God wanted me to participate. I could also sense I would have a major role even though I couldn't begin to imagine what God had in mind. I committed at that moment—sight unseen—to whatever the program required. I wanted what the Lord wanted. Early in the program I was quickly convicted that the First Place lifestyle was what the Lord wanted me to live the rest of my days. Three to four months into the program, I walked through my kitchen (past the scales) and I knew I had been set free from the bondage I'd been under so much of my life! It no longer mattered what I weighed or what size I wore. By giving up and surrendering control of my appetite and food choices to God, I received control from Him. I was no longer controlled by the lust of my flesh. It was no longer what I wanted but what He wanted and I firmly believe He wants me to follow the Live-It plan as is, to exercise, and to be in a daily personal relationship with Him through prayer and the Word. Through the nine commitments, I learned my problem was a spiritual problem. I'd never made the connection before, but food and appetite were false gods. Food separated me from God because I turned to it for comfort instead of to Him. I questioned Him—why did He make me this way? I didn't believe He could help me, which was evident in my decision in December 1994 to live

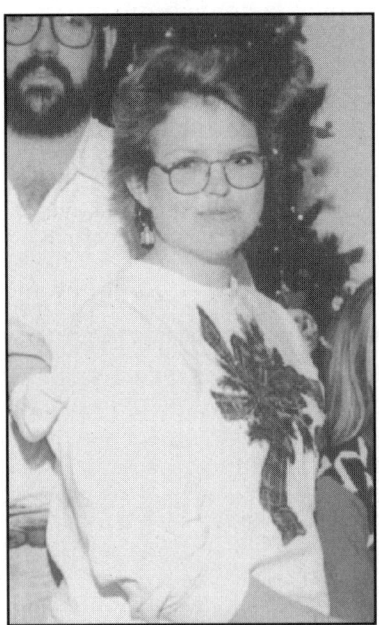

SHARON KING
BEFORE

the rest of my life overweight and out of control. Today I shudder when I think that I was willing to accept that defeated, unfulfilled lifestyle. Thank the Lord He doesn't give up on us even when we do. After choosing to be obedient in January 1995, I reached my lifetime goal in about seven months. I attended a First Place conference in Taylors, South Carolina and began leading classes. I've been privileged to witness lives being changed. The Lord is at work in Florence and surrounding areas. I've felt led to assist churches of different denominations organize classes, to share my testimony, to organize a leader's meeting within our association, to help organize a one-day conference for members within our area, to lead home groups and groups within local schools.

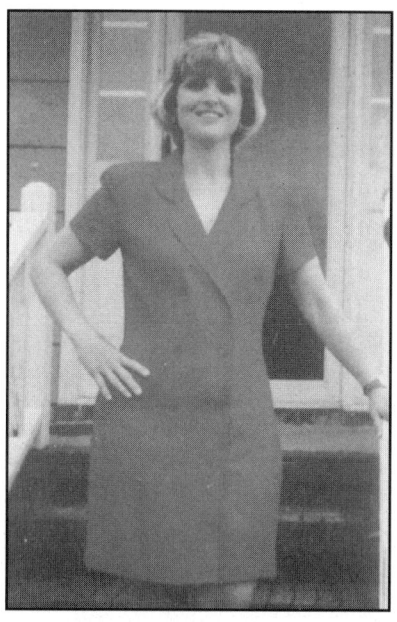

SHARON KING
AFTER

There are so many changes in my life in every area. I have truly been transformed by God. Words fail to describe the joy and new abundant life I know in Christ as I have discovered the last fruit of the Spirit—self-control. I thank God for the program and the first members who were obedient and committed to His work as well as the present First Place staff. Because of Him and them, I know my Lord and God as never before. To God be all the glory.

JULIE KUHN
Millport, Alabama

It all happened in October 1995. My husband had a job interview in West Virginia, and they wanted him to bring his wife. It was the first

FIRST PLACE

time in eighteen years that Doug and I had been anywhere without our boys. It was exciting, but I was the fattest I had been in my whole life. I didn't know what to wear because I didn't want to embarrass Doug, although he had never said anything about my weight. It wasn't him. I had a problem with how I looked. We went and had a good time, but I felt like a "fattening hog"

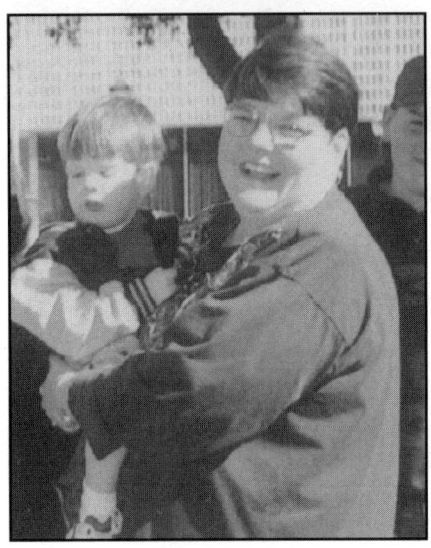

JULIE KUHN
BEFORE

In that old motel room in West Virginia, I decided I had to do something. But what? I sure didn't know. I had tried everything in the past. I could always lose weight, but it always came back.

In November, my friends and I went on our annual trip to Boaz Outlet Shopping. My friend Joyce Ann had on baggy jeans. I asked how much weight she had lost and she said, "I'm so excited, I've lost thirty pounds." Of course, I asked her how she did it. She began to explain that she had joined First Place in Vernon, Alabama. Joyce Ann was so excited about how God was helping her. She said they were starting a new session the week after Thanksgiving. She told me to call one of the leaders and talk to her. I couldn't wait to call. I called Sue. She was just as excited as Joyce Ann and had lost fifty pounds! I told her to put my name on the list.

The first week, I was really nervous because I have never been much of a Bible reader, and everyone else seemed to know a lot about the Bible. My Bible (actually it was my son's) looked brand new, and theirs were tattered and worn. Don't get me wrong, I was a Christian and a churchgoer, but still something was missing. I came home and read all my First Place information and did my first day's lesson. I felt

Personal Testimonies

closer to God already! It was so exciting that I could hardly wait until the next week.

Since that first week at First Place, I feel that I have grown spiritually and that my relationship with God has skyrocketed. My first "First Place Celebration" was on my fortieth birthday, and I had lost thirty-nine pounds. I felt like a new person "inside and out." I had never asked God to help me with my weight problem. I thought that He had more important things to do, but in First Place I learned that God cares about every aspect of my life. God loves me and He wants me to be healthy and happy. God and First Place have given me a new sort of confidence in *me*. The support and love that I have received from my First Place group has been overwhelming.

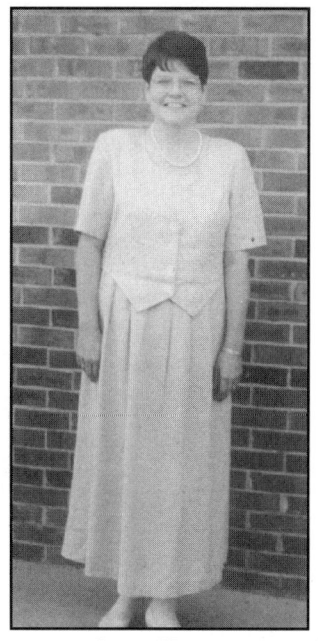

JULIE KUHN
AFTER

My husband and youngest son (my oldest son was in college) were going on a two-week Boy Scout trip, and this would give me the opportunity to spend some special time with my mother. I was so confident that I booked a cruise to the Bahamas for Mama and myself. By the time we set sail, I had lost fifty-six pounds and was not afraid to wear a bathing suit in public. We had a great time and the time I spent with my mother will be cherished forever.

As of this date, I have lost seventy-two pounds. I not only have a new wardrobe; I have a new attitude about life. I don't even think about First Place as a diet program. Losing weight is only the side effect of a program that has brought me closer to God and helped me to put Him in first place.

FIRST PLACE

FRANCES K. MIDDLEBROOKS
Texarkana, Texas

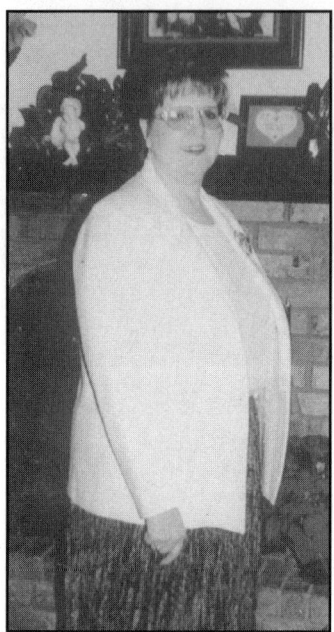

FRANCES MIDDLEBROOKS
BEFORE

I am approaching my second anniversary this month in First Place. My before and after pictures show a sixty-pound weight loss which I've been able to maintain for one year. I've also ended my twenty-year period of taking high blood pressure medicine. Diabetes runs in my family, and now I'm assured that I can take care of myself so that I won't have diabetes. The greatest blessing is that I'm able to share First Place with others through my church, in Texarkana, Arkansas.

As long as I can remember, I always had a weight problem. In high school, I made the basketball team, but my mom had to make my shorts. She did the best she could by adding the same trim of the uniforms so that I would not feel so out of place. As it happened, I had the whooping cough and I had to drop out of basketball. I was always the largest girl in the crowd. I loved graduation because my gown covered my faults. I tried every doctor's diet, every fad diet that came along. Have you ever tried the watermelon diet? Every other day you eat all the watermelon you want. Nothing else. I lost weight. I stayed in the bathroom! Once I did reach my goal weight, but I gained it back and more. I hated myself for being fat! I didn't have the willpower. I knew food wasn't what was wrong with me.

In fact, when I learned about First Place, I was weighing-in and leaving another weight loss program. I rarely stayed for the meetings. I was miserable. I lost weight, but I felt like I was pulling it off. My emotional

Personal Testimonies

needs were not being met. If First Place began in 1981, why did it take fourteen years for me to learn about it? I was desperate. In God's time a friend shared with me about First Place. I knew it was for me. I found freedom from insecurity, denial, and helplessness. I began trusting God to do a miracle on me. I had to do my part by being accountable to keep the First Place commitments. The exercise commitment was the most difficult, because I have a shoulder injury from a fall on a wet floor in January 1994. (One million people seemingly saw me fall. I was then at my peak weight.) Even walking would cause pain and discomfort. It seemed as if my pulse beat was in my shoulder. I was stagnated by fear. My doctor recommended surgery and I was terrified. Previous surgery on my foot had left lasting side effects that I still deal with. I was full of fear!

I had been successful losing the weight without the exercise. I was so enthused about First Place, I attended Fitness Week in Round Top, Texas, March 1996. Dr. Dick Couey lectured about nutrition and exercise. Of course, I was full of excuses why I could not participate in fitness testing. Dr. Couey's response was "get it fixed." It seemed so simple. He encouraged me to seek a specialist in a large city who performed only shoulder surgeries. The thought never occurred to me! My doctor referred me to an upper-extremities specialist in Dallas. On my first visit I knew I could trust the surgeon. I give God the glory because he placed me at Round Top to hear Dr. Couey and learn how fear had taken hold of me! I have recovered from the surgery and gone through physical therapy. Now I am exercising by walking at the track, and doing some floor exercises.

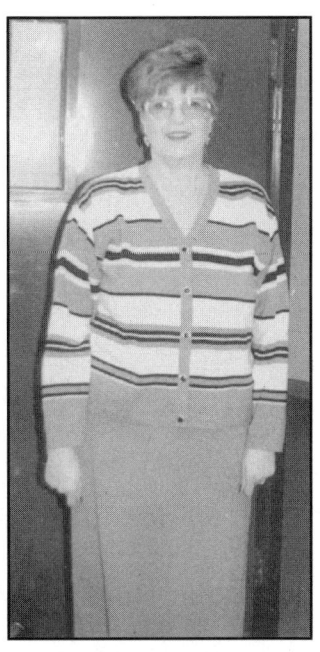

FRANCES MIDDLEBROOKS
AFTER

FIRST PLACE

I serve the Lord by being the First Place coordinator and leading a class at Trinity. Now we have four different groups including one that meets during the Sunday school hour. In First Place, God has blessed the lives of many through weight loss and a more personal relationship with Jesus that goes far beyond the figure on a scale. It's quite spectacular when I invite Jesus to share my "plate of food" and every aspect of my life. Thank God for First Place!

CAROLYN PONDER
Brandon, Mississippi

I began in First Place at my church, on July 5, 1995. I now consider this my Dependence Day, for after eating whatever I wanted at the church Independence Day celebration, I began the next day to learn to depend on Christ to take control of the physical things in my life. I no longer belong to Christ in the spiritual sense only; He has complete control of my life. Through Him I have lost sixty-five pounds and have maintained my weight with no trouble since September.

What freedom! I never knew that eating right and losing weight could be anything other than a struggle. Now I'm not controlled by food and cravings for food, but I use food as God intended— to keep my body healthy.

I now enjoy exercising like I never have before, although it had been a part of my routine for several years. I know that some exercise is better than none, but compared with what I can do now, it was nothing. I walk on the treadmill and do leg lifts/crunches and strength training on alternating days and I feel great! I'm fifty-six and feel better than I did at

CAROLYN PONDER
BEFORE

Personal Testimonies

twenty-six. I truly never really get tired. Sometimes I just go out and walk because I have so much energy. (And that's after a day of teaching first grade!)

Now I want to tell you about my First Place Group at First Presbyterian Day School in Jackson: We had our first meeting on Valentine's Day, 1996. Of the original group, most are still attending, and we have had some others join.

I have one friend who had already lost some weight and has lost sixty more pounds on First Place. She looks like a completely different person! I've taught with her for twenty years, and I'd forgotten what a beautiful lady she is physically as well as spiritually.

Two new members this last session have lost twenty and fifteen pounds respectively. They are just amazed at what First Place can do for them. The other members who have been in the group since the first or second session have lost anywhere from five to twenty pounds. Several really didn't need to lose more than a few pounds, but have stayed in the program because of the Bible study. It has been such a blessing to all of us!

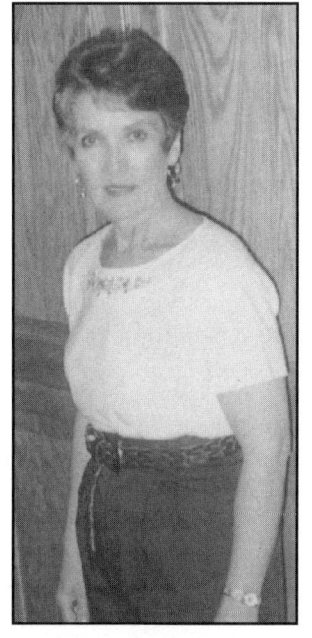

CAROLYN PONDER
AFTER

The parents of the children in our school have really noticed the change in many of the teachers. They have been very complimentary and supportive.

The parents of the children I teach have mentioned that they are pleased that I help encourage their children to make good food choices. My class knows which foods are healthy, and we have many good conversations over lunch about eating food that is good for our Temple.

I had never realized until I began First Place that I was limiting my ministry as a Christian teacher by being such a terrible physical role

FIRST PLACE

model. I truly feel that God is using the success He has given me to enrich the lives of the children I teach.

It's exciting to wait and see where God will take First Place next!

KATHIE SMITH
Davie, Florida

I have been married to Dick for thirteen years, and we have two children, Tommy, nine, and Melinda, six. I worked as a carrier for the U.S. Postal Service for ten years while trying to be a good wife and mother and still have time left to devote to God and my church. My life was a blur of trying to do everything but really doing little correctly. I kept up a good front most of the time but things were slipping out of control. I turned forty in November, but even before that I was fighting a losing battle with my weight, and I was tired all the time.

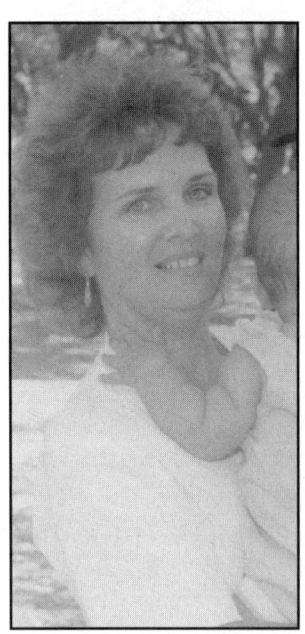

KATHIE SMITH
BEFORE

My husband and I had prayed for several years that I could quit my job and find something to do part-time at home so I could be here for our children, but every idea we came up with hit a dead end, until God finally showed us, through books and other ways, how we could make it on one income.

So I retired from the Post Office on Christmas Eve, and I thanked God for answering my long-time prayer request. I prayed that I would find a ministry that would fill the free time I had while my children were in school but still leaving me with flexibility so I could be there when they needed me. Right after the first of the year I began walking in the morning when I dropped the kids off at school, but

Personal Testimonies

I needed even more than that. I needed accountability.

I had heard of First Place from a few area churches and was interested, but I just didn't want to go to another church. I had begun walking once a week with my pastor's wife, Pam McCord, and mentioned this to her. She said she would also like to attend but wished it would come to our church one day. This is how, after much prayer, God led me to my friend, Mary Ann Rowe, who had worked with fitness and nutrition for fifteen years. First Place was brought to First Baptist Church of West Hollywood. After months of preparation, we began our first class with thirteen women.

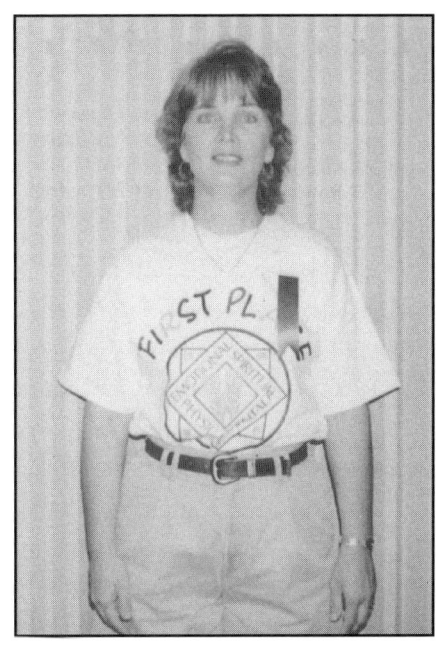

KATHIE SMITH
AFTER

This is my fifth week of being on the Live-It program, and I have lost eleven pounds. My husband is eating the same menu and has lost twelve pounds. My children are eating nutritious meals and snacks and liking it. I walk or do some form of exercise five times a week and I have so much energy, I feel better than I ever can remember feeling. I am already down a size, and it's even starting to get loose. I write about the physical changes but emotionally, mentally, and spiritually the changes are just as powerful in my life.

I am so excited about this program, and I love sharing that excitement with the ladies who are just beginning the program. I am so very grateful for First Place and to all of the people who have worked so hard on preparing it. Did you ever think that from this program's conception in 1981, people would still just be getting started and be just as excited in April 1997?

FIRST PLACE

KAY SMITH
First Place Associate Director
Houston, Texas

I was raised in the country and being a little overweight didn't seem like a problem. It became a big problem when I reached my teen years. I started my first diet with a doctor prescribing diet pills. It worked! The weight came off very fast and then I went back to eating all the good things I had been doing without. Now the problem was back and with a few extra pounds. I began at that early age a pattern that continued for twenty-five years—a constant yo-yo. I married and the weight problem increased after two children and years of diet pills and fad diets.

We spent thousands of dollars on my weight loss adventures and I lost weight with each thing I tried, but the weight was always back within a shorter time than it took to lose it. I would be successful for a time and then I would run out of willpower and eat something that I shouldn't and begin a binge. I would quit dieting for a time, eating everything I felt I had been deprived of. Even during the successful weeks I always had the thought, "I will get to my goal and then I can go back to eating all the things I want to eat." I had become very defensive about my weight, often even offended when people offered their advice or help. I had come to believe that this was my "cross to bear." I was destined to always be overweight.

I remember so well the Monday that I sat down in the empty sanctuary at my church and told God that I didn't want to live

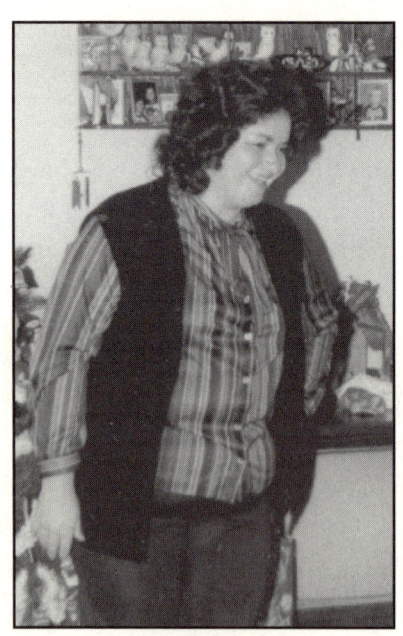

KAY SMITH
BEFORE

anymore. I felt completely helpless to overcome this tremendous problem in my life. I had truly hit bottom. That day I told God, "I give up. I am unable to control this area of my life." I believe that time alone in the sanctuary is one of the spiritual markers in my life. I was so aware of God's presence and of His assurance that this was not too big of a problem for Him. I went into the church office and spoke to a good friend. I was honest with her about my depression and I asked her if she had ever heard of any "Christian" weight loss program. She got me in touch with *First Place*.

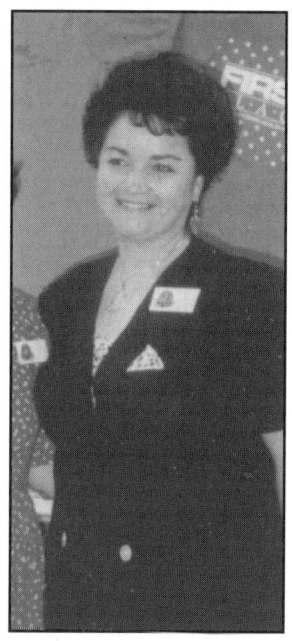

KAY SMITH
AFTER

Reluctantly I attended the orientation. I listened as each commitment was explained and thought, " I think I could do that." It was not a surprise to me to realize that I needed some discipline in my life. I felt such assurance that this was where God wanted me and the more I heard about the program, I believed that God had made it just for me. I did not lose a single pound at that orientation, but I felt like I had lost a hundred pounds. I did not understand how God was going to do this, but I believed He could. I had been given hope.

That night was only the beginning of a tremendous journey in my life. It has not been an easy journey. The weight loss of ninty pounds is fantastic, but it doesn't compare to the other blessings I have received. I never dreamed that I needed any emotional healing. I learned how much better relationships can be when you learn how to share emotional pain and joy. I was sure I didn't need any spiritual growth; I said my prayers every night. However First Place taught me how to have a personal daily relationship with Jesus. I began to be concerned about what I filled my mind with. God's Word became a personal letter that I wanted to spend more time reading. God's Word and the personal time spent with Him have given me the strength I need each day. One of the greatest blessings in my life is that the fear of gaining this weight back is gone. I have truly made a permanent lifestyle change; and I consider it my privilege to eat healthy and exercise. I also realize that you cannot fail *First Place*. I believe that the success is in the process.

I do not believe God caused me to be overweight. He took a weakness in my life and used it to draw me into a relationship with Him that is molding me into a servant He can use. He used it to give me His strength. One of my life verses is Philippians 1:6: "Being confident of this, that he who began a good work in you [Kay] will carry it on to completion until the day of Christ Jesus."

PAULA V. STACEY
Monroeville, Alabama

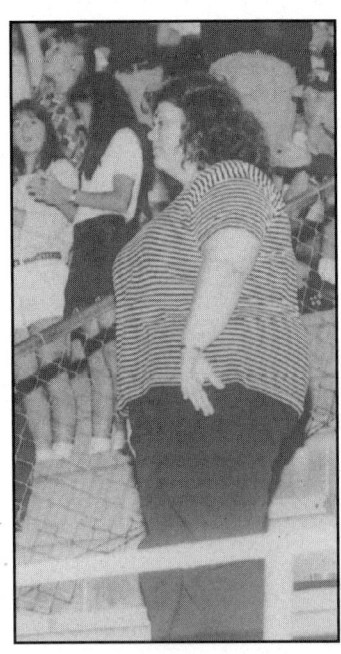

PAULA STACEY
BEFORE

I can't believe that I am writing this testimony, but it is due to God's empowerment and loving care. In May 1995, I began First Place in Monroeville. Was I apprehensive! I was scared, but I had reached the point that I was ready to do something about my weight. The first time I stepped on the scales, I weighted 295 pounds and wore a size 26. I was in terrible health. In fact, I really believe that I was about to die of a heart problem. I began the program and did it by the books (First Place and the Bible)! After the first week, I stepped on the scales, and I hadn't lost an ounce. I fell to pieces. But I kept on and began losing consistently. As I write this testimony, I have lost 140 pounds and I wear a size 10 or 12. I have lost over 100

Personal Testimonies

inches over the past 21 months. More importantly, I have grown so much spiritually. I have allowed God to empower me to control my eating and exercise habits. He has taught me discipline (the big D) in so many areas of my life. I am a changed person on the outside and inside. I am so grateful for God's provision of this program.

I am burdened with the testimony to encourage others to do First Place just as it is written. The success of the program lies in the nine commitments you make. I can honestly say that I have lived the First Place program because I believe if you are going to do something, do it right or do not do it at all! Each commitment is so important,

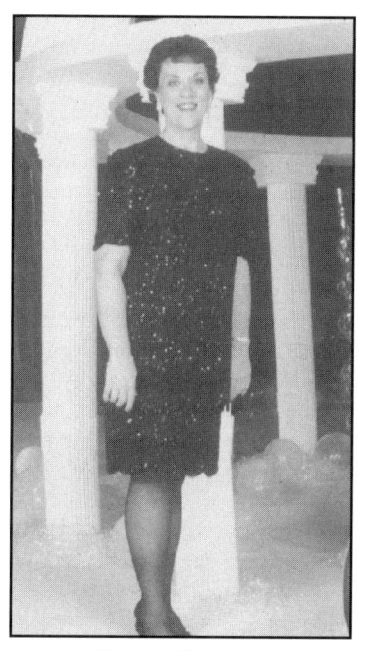

PAULA STACEY
AFTER

but I have to mention two of my favorites. First, the one that has meant the most to me is the memorizing of scripture. I remember thinking, "How can memorizing scripture help me lose weight? That's ridiculous!" But it did. It gave me encouragement and the ability to stay focused on the enormous task that lay ahead. The Scripture taught me that I can't, but God can (Phil. 4:13). Second, as a former couch potato, I can honestly say that I have really grown to love exercising. I can see and feel its benefits. I have learned that it releases stress and makes you feel good about yourself. It has become a natural part of my life—just like breathing. It's something I enjoy doing. It is a huge factor in my success in First Place.

I give praise to God for the staff of First Place (past and present) and their heeding of God's leading. I thank God for Peggy Vann (my Barnabas, my encourager) who found out about First Place and presented it to my church and became my first leader. I thank God for my pastor and my deacons who felt the importance of a Christian health program. I thank God for Scott Wilson, my second leader, who taught me so much about good nutrition and healthy cooking. I also thank God for all my friends in First Place and my church family who encouraged me as I strove toward the goal. You'll never know how much the calls, cards, and comments helped me stay the course (they still do)! I praise God for my family and their constant support, especially my son, Marcus, and my dad. Lastly and most importantly, I praise God for His intervention in my life through First Place. I worked hard, prayed hard, and gave it to God, and God worked a miracle! He can do it for you too—if you give Him First Place!

PAT STOKES
Camden, South Carolina

I first heard about First Place in September 1996. I found the concept of weight loss and Bible study together very interesting. I needed to lose twenty-five pounds, so I seriously considered starting a program in our church and even mentioned it during one of our women's meetings. Instead of a pursuing the idea any further, I pushed the thought of the program aside because I didn't have time to attend a First Place class, much less lead one. I work full-time and was a full-time college student in the evenings. I had waited a long time to go back to college to finish my teaching degree. This was my time and I didn't want anything to interfere with *my* plans. It seemed that more often than I wanted, I would hear or read something concerning First Place. God was convicting me to start a program at our church. Each time I

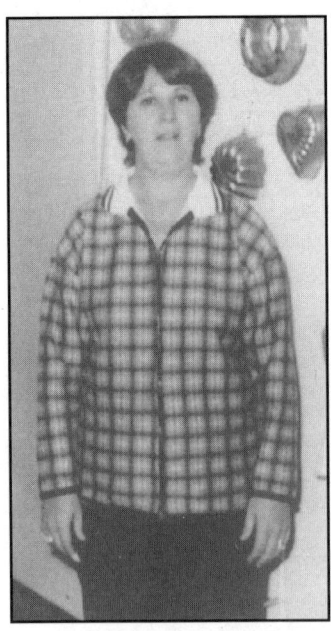

PAT STOKES
BEFORE

Personal Testimonies

would convince myself that I didn't have time and besides, I was the pastor's wife and I did plenty in the church already.

One day while I was at work, a young lady came into my office to talk about taking some courses through the adult education program (that's where I work). After a few minutes I realized I knew this person but just couldn't put my finger on from where. She turned out to be the wife of the former pastor of the church we are currently serving. I had met her one time when her husband had come back to preach the homecoming message. Of course we had a lot to talk about, but all she wanted to talk about was the First Place program that was going on in their church. She went on and on about the program, and I just didn't want to hear it. Every time I heard the words First Place, I would come under conviction about starting a program at our church. This young lady came to my office to chat every day for two weeks—every day she told me something else wonderful about their First Place program. Finally I was under so much conviction, one year after first hearing about First Place, I told God OK. I quit college. I started talking and contacting other churches and leaders to learn all I could about the First Place program. I know in my heart that God used a fellow Christian and pastor's wife to be a part of that convicting power to help me make my decision.

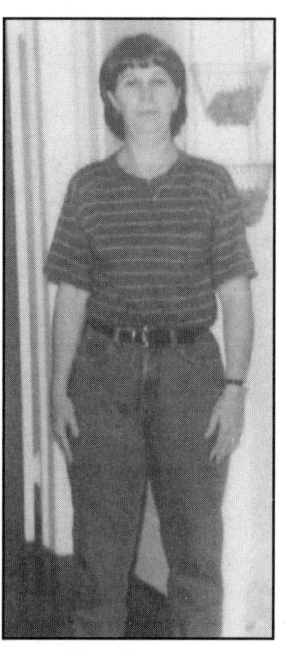

PAT STOKES
AFTER

I told my husband that I wanted God off my back and that I was going to lead a First Place group in the church. I also told him that I knew there wouldn't be two people to join, because we are a small rural church. Secretly I was hoping that no one would join so I could tell God I had done what He wanted me to do and it didn't fly. I could go back to college to do what I wanted. I announced the First Place program in church, and within a week sixteen people told me they were interested, some from in the church and some from outside of the church.

I cannot tell you how God has blessed my life and others through First Place. Through this program not only has the weight come off of myself and others, but some people who had drifted away from God are back in the church and working for His glory. We are now finishing a second session that meets on Sunday nights, and I started another group that meets on Wednesday night. Our Sunday school director wants to start a class during Sunday school and I even have had other churches ask me to conduct a class at their church. I am so glad I listened to God. I have reached my goal weight, and as I watch others lose weight and grow spiritually it truly makes me joyful.

Through First Place, God has shown me that my aspiration to be a teacher has been fulfilled. It isn't the classroom that I thought I would be in, but it is the classroom God wants me in.

So many people in our town who have benefited from this wonderful program. First Place is growing by leaps and bounds in our area.

CAROL J. WHITE
Fort Walton Beach, Florida

I have tried just about every diet in existence, going up and down in my weight over the years. I even tried the fad diet that required fasting for a week, 1,000 calories the next, and fasting again. I even took the drastic step of having my stomach stapled, which worked for a while, but I finally had given up on trying to keep the weight off until God brought my attention to First Place. The First Place orientation was scheduled to be given on the second floor of my church and even that was probably for a reason. My knees hurt with every step and I realized that if I did not lose weight I might not be able to walk in another few years, much less climb stairs.

I started First Place in August of 1995 at the age of 59 and weighing 267 pounds. I had a wonderful leader, Tina Ward, who encouraged me as she led the group. The daily Bible study, scripture reading, and

Personal Testimonies

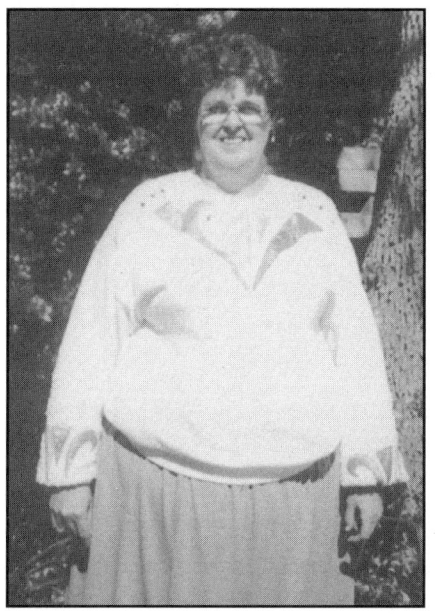

CAROL WHITE
BEFORE

prayer each morning was a real inspiration. God gave me the strength and courage to face each day and convicted me that my eating habits were sinful and that I needed to change. I went sugar-free the first session and I can tell you that only God could do that with me.

I have now lost ninty-two pounds and kept it off. What a joy it is just to be able to walk better, climb stairs easier. Even getting up out of my chair is a reminder of how good God is when we put Him in first place.

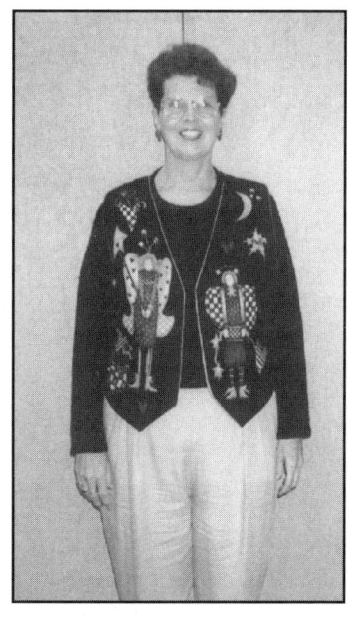

CAROL WHITE
AFTER

My weight loss has been an excellent way to witness for my precious Lord as people ask how I was able to get the weight off. It is a joy to share my witness of the all-powerful God as He used the First Place program to get my attention.

The first session I was in had eight members and the one just completed had sixty, including some men. I have led two sessions myself in Fort Walton Beach and have enjoyed all aspects of the program and feel each is equally important to those wishing to lose weight. I personally am grateful to God and First Place.

FIRST PLACE

I could not categorize my testimony since no one aspect of the program is more important to me than the others. I feel the sharing of our experiences, Bible study, prayer, and just general good support in the program are all important, and those who don't do all of them don't do well. My experience says you have to commit in all aspects if you are to succeed.

APPENDIX B

Live-It Food Exchanges

Women start with no less than 1,200. Men no less than 1,500.

Food Exchanges	Calories Per Day									
	1,200	1,400	1,500	1,600	1,800	2,000	2,200	2,400	2,600	2,900
	Number of Exchanges									
Morning										
Lean Meat Exchange	1	1	1	1	2	2	2	2	2	2
Bread Exchange	1	1	2	2	3	3	4	4	4	5
Fruit Exchange	1	1	1	1	1	1	1	2	2	2
Milk Exchange	1	1	1	1	1	1	1	1	1	1
Fat Exchange	1	1	1	1	1	1	1	2	2	3
Midday										
Lean Meat Exchange	2	2	2	2	2	2	2	2	2	2
Bread Exchange	2	2	2	3	3	4	4	5	5	5
Vegetable Exchange*	1	1	1	1	1	1	1	2	2	2
Fruit Exchange	1	1	1	1	1	1	1	1	1	3
Milk Exchange	½	½	½	½	½	½	½	½	1	1
Fat Exchange	1	1	1	1	1	2	3	3	3	3
Evening										
Lean Meat Exchange	2	2	2	2	3	3	3	3	3	3
Bread Exchange	2	4	4	4	4	4	4	4	5	5
Vegetable Exchange*	1	1	1	2	2	2	2	2	3	3
Fruit Exchange	1	1	1	1	1	1	2	2	2	2
Milk Exchange	½	½	½	½	½	½	½	½	1	1
Fat Exchange	1	1	2	2	2	3	4	4	4	4

FIRST PLACE

% Carbohydrate	55	55	55	55	55	55	55	55	55	55
% Protein	20	20	20	20	20	20	20	20	20	20
% Fat	25	25	25	25	25	25	25	25	25	25

Vegetables listed are a daily minimum. You may eat additional exchanges from the Vegetables List, preferably raw.

Pregnant and nursing mothers—consult your doctor. Artificial sweeteners are not recommended.

FOOD GROUPS
MEAL PLANNING WITH EXCHANGES

The six Exchange Lists, or food groups (listed below), were developed to aid in menu planning for First Place. The individual diet plan prescribed by a physician and/or registered dietitian indicates the number of servings from each food group that should be eaten at each meal and snack. All the foods within a group contain approximately the same amount of nutrients and calories per serving, which means that one serving of a food from the starch list may be exchanged (or substituted) for one serving of any other item in the starch list. The chart below shows the amount of nutrients and number of calories in one serving from each food group. Each food group is important. If for any reason you cannot or choose not to eat from a particular food group, consult with a physician or nutritionist to insure proper nutrition.

Exchange List	Carbohydrate (grams)	Protein (grams)	Fat (grams)	Calories
Starch/Bread	15	3	trace	80
Meat				
Lean	—	7	3	55
Medium-fat	—	7	5	75
High-fat	—	7	8	100
Vegetable	5	2	—	25

Live-It Food Exchanges

Exchange List	Carbohydrate (grams)	Protein (grams)	Fat (grams)	Calories
Fruit	15	—	—	60
Milk				
Skim	12	8	trace	90
Low-fat	12	8	5	120
Whole	12	8	8	150
Fat	—	—	5	45

EXCHANGE LISTS
BREAD LIST

Each item on the *Bread* list contains approximately 15 grams of carbohydrate, 3 grams of protein, a trace of fat, and 80 calories. A trace of fat is less than 1 gram. Bread products containing 2 or 3 grams of fat will count 1 bread + ½ fat. If the product contains 4 or 5 grams of fat, it counts as 1 bread + 1 fat. When choosing cereal, check the nutritional information carefully for grams of fat and sugar. Simple sugar will be listed at the bottom, 4 grams = 1 teaspoon of sugar. We recommend anything below 5 grams. Check to see if the cereal is a good source of fiber. Fiber counts vary from 0 grams to 13+ per serving. The amount of sugar varies with each cereal. When you have eaten cereal equaling 80 calories, you have eaten one bread exchange. Whole grain products average about 2 grams of fiber per serving. Some foods are higher in fiber. Those foods that contain 3 or more grams of fiber per serving are identified with a * symbol.

You can choose starch exchanges from any of the items on this list. If you want to eat a starch food that is not on the list, the general rule is that:

½ cup of cereal, grain, or pasta is one serving,
1 ounce of a bread product is one serving.

FIRST PLACE

CEREALS, GRAINS, AND PASTA

Bran cereals, concentrated* (such as Bran Buds, All Bran)	⅓ cup
Bran cereals, flaked*	½ cup
Bulgur (cooked)	½ cup
Cooked cereals	½ cup
Grapenuts	3 tablespoons
Grits (cooked)	½ cup
Other ready to eat unsweetened cereals	¾ cup
Pasta (cooked)	½ cup
Puffed cereal	1½ cups
Rice, white or brown (cooked)	⅓ cup
Shredded wheat	½ cup

DRIED BEANS, PEAS, AND LENTILS

Beans and peas (cooked),* such as pinto, kidney, white, split, black-eyed	⅓ cup
Lentils (cooked)*	⅓ cup
Baked beans*	¼ cup

ALTERNATIVE EXCHANGE

Beans, peas, and lentils*	1 cup = 2 breads
1 lean meat	

*3 grams or more of fiber per serving

STARCHY VEGETABLES

Corn*	½ cup
Corn on cob,* 6 inches long	1 ear
Hominy	½ cup
Lima beans*	½ cup
Peas, green* (canned or frozen)	½ cup
Plantain*	½ cup
Potato, baked	1 small (3 ounces)
Potato, mashed	½ cup

Live-It Food Exchanges

Pumpkin	¾ cup
Squash, winter (acorn, butternut)	¾ cup
Yam, sweet potato, plain	⅓ cup

BREAD

Bagel	½ (1 ounce)
Bread sticks, crisp, 4 inches long x ½-inch	2 (⅔ ounce)
Croutons, low-fat	1 cup
English muffin	½
Frankfurter or hamburger bun	½ (1 ounce)
Pita, 6 inches across	½
Plain roll, small	1 (1 ounce)
Raisin, unfrosted	1 slice (1 ounce)
Rye, pumpernickel*	1 slice (1 ounce)
Tortilla, corn, 6 inches across	1
Tortilla, flour, 6 inches across	1 + ½ fat
White (including French, Italian)	1 slice (1 ounce)
Whole wheat	1 slice (1 ounce)
"Diet" bread (40 calories each)	2 slices

CRACKERS AND SNACKS

Matzoh	¾ ounce
Melba toast	5 slices
Oyster crackers	24
Popcorn (popped, no fat added)	3 cups
Pretzels	¾ ounce
Rice cakes	2 regular, 6 mini
Rye crisp, 2 inches x 3½ inches	4
Saltine-type crackers	6
Whole wheat crackers, no fat added (crisp breads, such as Finn, Kavli, Wasa)	2-4 slices (¾ ounce)

*3 grams or more of fiber per serving

FIRST PLACE

STARCH FOODS PREPARED WITH FAT

(Count as 1 starch/bread serving, plus 1 fat serving)

Biscuit, 2½ inches across	1
Chow mein noodles	½ cup
Cornbread, 2-inch cube	1 (2 ounces)
Cracker, round butter type	6
French fried potatoes, 2 inches to 3½ inches long	10 (1-½ ounces)
Muffin, plain, small	1
Pancake, 4 inches across	2
Rolls, butter style	1
Stuffing, bread (prepared)	¼ cup
Taco shell, 6 inches across	1
Tortilla chips	5
Waffle, five-by-one-half inch (Count as 1 starch/bread and 2 fat exchanges)	1
Corn chips	1 ounce
Croissant	1 small, 1 ounce
Potato chips	1 ounce
Baking chocolate	1 ounce

Miscellaneous Bread

The following are equivalent to one Bread Exchange, although many are not as nutritious as other selections from the Bread Exchange group.

Barbecue sauce	¼ cup
Barley, dry	1½ tablespoon
Bran, raw unprocessed	½ cup
Bread crumbs, dried	2 tablespoons
Catsup	¼ cup
Chili sauce	¼ cup
Cocoa	5 tablespoons
Cornmeal	2½ tablespoons

Live-It Food Exchanges

Cornstarch	2 tablespoons
Flour	2½ tablespoons or 1 cup = 5 breads
Malt, dry	1 tablespoon or ⅔ ounce
Tapioca	2 tablespoons
Tomato paste	6 tablespoons
Tomato sauce	1 cup
Wheat germ*	3 tablespoons
Yogurt, frozen nonfat	3 ounce serving

* 3 grams or more of fiber per serving

MEAT LIST

Each serving of the *meat* and *meat substitutes* on this list contain about *7 grams of protein*. The amount of fat and number of calories vary, depending on what kind of meat or substitute you choose. The meat list is divided into three parts based on the amount of fat and calories: lean meat, medium-fat meat, and high-fat meat. One ounce (one meat exchange) of each includes:

	Carbohydrate (grams)	Protein (grams)	Fat (grams)	Calories
Lean	0	7	3	55
Medium-fat	0	7	5	75
High-fat	0	7	8	100

You are encouraged to use more lean and medium-fat meat, poultry, and fish in your meal plan. This will help decrease your fat intake, which may help decrease your risk for heart disease. The items from the high-fat group are high in saturated fat, cholesterol, and calories. You should limit your choices from the high-fat group to three (3) times per week. Meat and substitutes do not contribute any fiber to your meal plan.

FIRST PLACE

LEAN MEAT AND SUBSTITUTES

Count as 1 meat exchange

Beef	USDA Good or Choice grades of lean beef, such as round, sirloin, and flank steak; tenderloin; and *chipped beef	1 ounce
Pork	Lean pork, such as fresh ham; canned, cured, or boiled ham, *Canadian bacon, *tenderloin	1 ounce
Veal	All cuts are lean except for veal cutlets (ground or cubed). Examples of lean veal are chops and roasts.	1 ounce
Poultry	Chicken, turkey, Cornish hen (without skin)	1 ounce
Fish	All fresh and frozen fish	1 ounce
	Crab, lobster, scallops, shrimp, clams* (fresh or canned in water)	2 ounces
	Oysters	6 medium
	Tuna* (canned in water)	1/4 cup
	Herring (uncreamed or smoked)	1 ounce
	Sardines (canned)	2 medium
Game	Venison, rabbit, squirrel	1 ounce
	Pheasant, duck, goose (without skin)	1 ounce
Cheese	Any cottage cheese	1/4 cup
	Grated parmesan	2 tablespoons
	Diet cheese* (with less than 55 calories per ounce, 1 gram of fat or less)	
	Fat-free cream cheese	1 ounce
Other	95 percent fat-free luncheon meat, (1 gram fat or less)	1 ounce
	Egg whites	3 whites
	Egg substitutes with less than 55 calories per 1/4 cup	1/4 cup

*400 milligrams or more of sodium per serving

Live-It Food Exchanges

MEDIUM-FAT MEAT AND SUBSTITUTES

Count 1 meat + ½ fat

Beef	Most beef products fall into this category. Examples are: all ground beef, roast (rib, chuck, rump), steak (cubed, Porterhouse, T-bone) and meatloaf.	1 ounce
Pork	Most pork products fall into this category. Examples are: chops, loin roast, Boston butt, cutlets.	1 ounce
Lamb	Most lamb products fall into this category. Examples are: chops, leg, and roast.	1 ounce
Veal	Cutlet (ground or cubed, unbreaded)	1 ounce
Poultry	Chicken (with skin), domestic duck or goose (well-drained of fat), ground turkey	1 ounce
Fish	Tuna* (canned in oil and drained)	¼ cup
	Salmon* (canned)	¼ cup
Cheese	Skim or part-skim milk cheeses such as:	
	Ricotta	¼ cup
	Mozzarella	1 ounce
	Diet cheese* (with 56-80 calories per ounce)	1 ounce
Other	Luncheon meat* (2 or 3 grams of fat)	1 ounce
	Egg (high cholesterol; limit 3 per week)	1 egg
	Egg substitutes with 56-80 calories per ¼ cup	¼ cup
	Tofu (2½ inches by 2¾ inches by 1 inch)	4 ounces
	Liver, heart, kidney, sweetbreads (high in cholesterol)	1 ounce

*400 milligrams or more of sodium per serving

FIRST PLACE

HIGH-FAT MEAT AND SUBSTITUTES

Count as 1 meat + 1 fat

Remember, these items are high in saturated fat, cholesterol, and calories, and should be used only three (3) times per week

Beef	Most USDA Prime cuts of beef, such as ribs, corned beef*	1 ounce
Pork	Spareribs, ground pork, pork sausage* (patty or link)	1 ounce
Lamb	Patties (ground lamb)	1 ounce
Fish	Any fried fish product	1 ounce
Cheese	All regular cheeses* such as American, Blue, Cheddar, Monterey, Swiss	1 ounce
Other	Luncheon meats* such as bologna, salami, pimiento loaf	1 ounce
	Sausage* such as Polish, Italian	1 ounce
	Knockwurst, smoked	1 ounce
	Bratwurst*	1 ounce
	Frankfurter* (turkey or chicken)	1 frank
	Peanut butter (contains unsaturated fat)	1 tablespoon

Count as 1 meat + 2 fat

	Frankfurter* (beef, pork, or combination)	1 frank

VEGETABLE LIST

Each vegetable serving on this list contains about 5 grams of carbohydrate, 2 grams of protein, and 25 calories. Vegetables contain 2-3 grams of dietary fiber. Two vegetable servings per day are the minimum amounts needed. Three to four vegetable servings are encouraged.

Vegetables are a good source of vitamins and minerals. Fresh and frozen vegetables have more vitamins and less added salt. Rinsing canned vegetables will remove excess salt.

Live-It Food Exchanges

Unless otherwise noted, the serving size for vegetables (one vegetable exchange) is:

½ cup of cooked vegetable
    or vegetable juice
1 cup of raw vegetables

VEGETABLE LIST

- Artichoke (½ medium)
- Asparagus
- Bamboo shoots
- Beans (green, wax, Italian)
- Bean sprouts
- Beets
- Broccoli
- Brussels sprouts
- Cabbage, cooked
- Carrots
- Carrot juice (¼ cup)
- Cauliflower
- Eggplant
- Greens (collard, mustard, turnip)
- Kohlrabi
- Leeks
- Mushrooms, cooked
- Okra
- Onions
- Pea pods
- Peppers (green)
- Pimento (3 oz.)
- Rutabaga
- Sauerkraut*
- Shallots (4 tablespoons)
- Snow peas
- Spinach, cooked
- Summer squash (crookneck)
- Tomato (one large)
- Tomato*/vegetable juice
- Turnips
- Water chestnuts
- Zucchini, cooked

*400 milligrams or more of sodium per serving

FREE VEGETABLES

Raw, 1 cup

- Alfalfa sprouts
- Bok Choy
- Cabbage
- Celery
- Chinese Cabbage
- Green onion
- Hot peppers
- Lettuce
- Mushrooms
- Parsley

FIRST PLACE

Cilantro
Cress, garden
Cucumber
Endive
Escarole

Radishes
Romaine
Spinach
Watercress
Zucchini

COMBINING VEGETABLE PROTEINS

Proper combining of plant proteins at any one meal can create a complete protein, supplying sufficient amino acids to the meal. To have meatless meals with the right amount and kind of protein, combine any food in Column I with food from Column II. The correct exchange will depend on the food chosen. Count each combination according to exchange guidelines. For example, if you combine beans and rice: $1/3$ cup rice = 1 bread, $1/3$ cup beans = 1 bread. An egg is still 1 meat and $1/2$ fat. When combining vegetables, if you are choosing to eliminate the meat exchange on your fact sheet, please check with your physician or dietician to adjust your exchange to insure proper nutrition.

Column I	Column II
Legumes	
Beans: aduki, black, broad or Fava, cranberry beans, garbanzo, (chick peas), Great Northern,	Grains Seeds and nuts Nonfat and low-fat dairy products
lima, marrow, mung, navy, pea, pinto, soy, white.	Eggs or egg substitutes
Peas:	
split blackeye (cow), field	
Lentils	
Textured vegetable protein	Tofu (soybean curd)
Grains	
Whole Grains: barley, buckwheat, corn	Legumes

Live-It Food Exchanges

oats, rice, rye triticale

Grain Products: bran, breads, bulgur, cereals, lowfat crackers, cornbread, flour, groats, Kasha, macaroni, millet (cracked wheat or couscous), pasta, popcorn, wheat germ, tortillas

Nuts
 almonds, beechnuts, brazil nuts, filberts, peanuts, peanut butter,

 pecans, pinenuts (pignolia), walnuts

Seeds
 Pumpkin, sesame, squash, sunflower

Eggs
 egg substitutes
 egg whites
 whole egg

Dairy Products
 nonfat or $1/2$ percent low-fat milk
 skim or low-fat buttermilk
 nonfat or low-fat yogurt
  low-fat cheese

Nonfat or low-fat dairy products
Eggs or egg substitutes

Legumes
Nonfat or low-fat dairy products
Eggs or egg substitutes

Grains
Legumes
Nuts and seeds

Refer to individual Exchange Group for the portion size.
Starchy vegetables such as corn, peas, and potatoes are found on the Starch/Bread List.

FIRST PLACE

FRUIT LIST

Each item on the Fruit List contains about 15 grams of carbohydrate and 60 calories. Fresh, frozen, and dry fruits have about 2 grams of fiber per serving. Fruit juices contain very little dietary fiber.

The carbohydrate and calorie content for a fruit serving are based on the usual serving of the most commonly eaten fruits. Use fresh fruits or fruits frozen or canned without sugar added. Whole fruit is more filling than fruit juice and may be a better choice for those who are trying to lose weight. Unless otherwise noted, the serving size for one fruit serving is:

½ cup of fresh fruit or fruit juice
¼ cup of dried fruit

FRESH, FROZEN, AND UNSWEETENED CANNED FRUIT

Apple (raw, 2 inches across)	1 apple, 4 ounces
Applesauce (unsweetened)	½ cup
Apricots (medium, raw) or	4 apricots
Apricots (canned)	½ cup, or 4 halves, 4 ounces
Banana (9 inches long)	½ banana, 3 ounces
Blackberries* (raw)	¾ cup
Blueberries* (raw)	¾ cup
Boysenberries	¾ cup
Cantaloupe (5 inches across)	⅓ melon, or 7 ounces
(cubes)	1 cup
Caranbola (starfruit)	3, or 7½ ounce
Cherries (large, raw)	12 cherries, or 3½ ounce
Cherries (canned)	½ cup
Crab apples	¾ cup, or 2¾ ounces
Dewberries	¾ cup, or 3 ounces
Figs (raw, 2 inches across)	2 figs, or 3 ounces
Fruit cocktail (canned)	½ cup
Goose berries	1 cup, or 5 ounces
Grapefruit (medium)	½ grapefruit
Grapefruit (segments)	¾ cup

Live-It Food Exchanges

Grapes (small)	15 grapes
Honeydew melon (medium) (cubes)	1/8 melon 1 cup
Kiwi (large)	1 kiwi, or 3¼ ounces
Kumquats	4 medium, or 3½ ounces
Mandarin oranges	¾ cup
Mango (small)	½ mango, or 3 ounces
Mulberries	1 cup, or 5 ounces
Nectarine* (1½ inches across)	1 nectarine, or 5 ounces
Orange (2½ inches across)	1 orange, or 6½ ounces
Papaya	1 cup, or 8 ounces
Passion Fruit	4, or 4 ounces
Peach (2¾ inches across)	1 peach, or ¾ cup
Peaches (canned)	½ cup, or 2 halves
Pear	½ large, or 1 small
Pears (canned)	½ cup, or 2 halves
Persimmon (medium, native)	2 persimmons
Pineapple (raw)	¾ cup
Pineapple (canned)	⅓ cup
Plum (raw, 2 inches across)	2 plums, or 5 ounces
Pomegranate*	½ pomegranate
Raspberries* (raw)	1 cup, or 3¾ ounces
Strawberries* (raw, whole)	1¼ cups, or 5½ ounces
Tangerine (2½ inches across)	2 tangerines, or 6½ ounces
Watermelon (cubes)	1¼ cups

DRIED FRUIT

Apples*	4 rings, or ¾ ounce
Apricots*	7 halves, or ¾ ounce
Dates	2½ medium
Figs*	1½
Prunes*	3 medium, or 1 ounce
Raisins	2 tablespoons, or ¾ ounce

*3 or more grams of fiber per serving

FIRST PLACE

FRUIT JUICE

Apple juice/cider	½ cup
Cranberry juice cocktail	⅓ cup
Grapefruit juice	½ cup
Grape juice	⅓ cup
Lemon juice (fresh, not concentrate)	1 cup
Lime juice	1 cup
Nectar:	½ cup, or 4 ounces
Apricot	
Papaya	
Pear	
Peach	
Orange juice	½ cup
Orange juice, frozen concentrate	2 tablespoons, or 1 ounce
Pineapple juice	½ cup
Prune juice	⅓ cup

MILK LIST

Each serving of milk or milk products on this list contains about 12 grams of carbohydrate and 8 grams of protein. The amount of fat in milk is measured in percent (%) of butterfat. The calories vary, depending on what kind of milk you choose. The list is divided into three parts based on the amount of fat and calories: skim/very low-fat milk, low-fat milk, and whole milk. One serving (one milk exchange) of each of these includes:

	Carbohydrate (grams)	Protein (grams)	Fat (grams)	Calories
Skim/very low-fat	12	8	trace	90
Low-fat	12	8	5	120
Whole	12	8	8	150

Milk is the body's main source of calcium, the mineral needed for growth and repair of bones. Yogurt also is a good source of calcium.

Live-It Food Exchanges

Yogurt and many dry or powdered milk products have different amounts of fat. If you have questions about a particular item, read the label to find out the fat and calorie content.

Milk is good to drink, but it can also be added to cereal and to other foods. Many tasty dishes, such as sugar-free pudding, are made with milk. Add variety to plain yogurt by mixing with one of your fruit servings. In many recipes, such as corn bread or muffins, you can substitute yogurt for oil. Yogurt is good added to sugar-free jello. For individuals who believe they cannot tolerate milk products, many products are on the market for people who suffer from lactose intolerance. Many of these people do fine eating dairy yogurt. A person who cannot tolerate any dairy products should see his or her physician to adjust personal exchanges.

SKIM AND VERY LOW-FAT MILK

One Exchange = 1 milk

Skim milk	1 cup
$1/2$ percent milk	1 cup
1 percent milk	1 cup
Low-fat buttermilk	1 cup
Evaporated skim milk	$1/2$ cup
Dry nonfat milk	$1/3$ cup
Nonfat dairy yogurt	8 ounces

LOW-FAT MILK

One Exchange = 1 milk +1 fat

$1 1/2$ percent milk	1 cup
2 percent milk	1 cup
Plain low-fat yogurt (with added nonfat milk solids)	8 ounces

WHOLE MILK

One Exchange = 1 milk + 2 fat

The whole milk group has much more fat per serving than the skim and low-fat groups. Whole milk has more than $3 1/4$ percent but-

FIRST PLACE

terfat. Try to limit your choices from the whole milk group as much as possible.

Whole milk	1 cup
Evaporated whole milk	½ cup
Whole plain yogurt	8 ounces

FAT LIST

Each serving on the Fat List contains about 5 grams of fat and 45 calories The foods on the Fat List contain mostly fat, although some items may also contain a small amount of protein. All fats are high in calories and should be carefully measured. Everyone should modify fat intake by eating unsaturated fats instead of saturated fats. The sodium content of these foods vary widely. Check the label for sodium information.

UNSATURATED FATS

Avocado	⅛ medium
Margarine	1 teaspoon
Margarine, diet*	1 tablespoon
Mayonnaise	1 teaspoon
Mayonnaise, reduced calorie*	1 tablespoon
Nuts and seeds:	
Almonds, dry roasted	6 whole
Cashews, dry roasted	1 tablespoon
Pecans	2 whole
Peanuts	20 small or 10 large
Walnuts	2 whole
Other nuts	1 tablespoon
Seeds, pine nuts, sunflower (without shells)	1 tablespoon
Pumpkin seeds	2 teaspoons
Oil (corn, cottonseed, safflower, soybean, sunflower, olive, peanut)	1 teaspoon
Olives*	10 small or 5 large
Salad dressing, mayonnaise-type	2 teaspoons

(Two tablespoons of low-calorie salad dressing is a free food.)

Live-It Food Exchanges

*If more than one or two servings are eaten, these foods have 400 milligrams or more of sodium

SATURATED FATS

Not Recommended for Use

Butter	1 teaspoon
Bacon*	1 slice
Chitterlings	½ ounce
Coconut, shredded	2 tablespoons
Coffee whitener, liquid	2 tablespoons
Coffee whitener, powder	4 teaspoons
Cream (light, coffee, table)	2 tablespoons
Cream, sour	2 tablespoons
Cream (heavy, whipping)	1 tablespoon
Cream cheese	1 tablespoon
Cream cheese, lite	2 tablespoons
Half-and-half	3 tablespoons
Salt pork*	¼ ounce
Sour cream	2 tablespoons
Whipping cream	1 tablespoon
Meat fat	1 teaspoon
Meat drippings	1 teaspoon
Chocolate (1 oz.)	1 bread, 2 fats

*If more than one or two servings are eaten, these foods have 400 mg. or more of sodium. If you choose a fat-free product normally listed under the fats category, limit serving to 20 calories or less.

FREE FOODS

The items on this list are very low in calories. They also contain few if any nutrients, Limit these free items to a total of 20 calories per day. Many of the foods or drinks listed contain sugar substitutes. First Place recommends "moderation" in using sugar substitutes.

FIRST PLACE

Drinks:
Bouillon or broth without fat
Bouillon (low-sodium)
Carbonated drinks, sugar-free
Carbonated water
Club soda
Cocoa powder, unsweetened (1 tbsp.)
Coffee/tea
Drink mixes, sugar-free
Tonic water, sugar-free

Fruit:
Cranberries, unsweetened (½ cup)
Rhubarb, unsweetened (½ cup)

Condiments:
Catsup (1 tbsp.)
Horseradish
Mustard
Pickles, dill or unsweetened
Fat-free margarine
Fat-free sour cream
Taco sauce (1 tbsp.)
Vinegar

Sugar substitutes:
Gelatin, sugar-free
Gum, sugar-free
Jam / Jelly, sugar-free or All Fruit (2 tsp.)

Sweet Substitutes:
Pancake syrup, sugar-free (1-2 tbsp.)
Sugar substitutes, saccharin, aspartame

Nonstick pan spray or vegetable cooking spray

Seasonings also are considered free foods, and they can be very helpful in making food taste better. However, be careful of how much sodium you use. Read the label and choose seasonings that do not contain sodium or salt.

*Recommended sodium intake is 3,000 milligrams per day

APPENDIX C
Fact Sheet Information

The First Place Fact Sheet is used to record everything that you eat for an entire week. You will begin a new Fact Sheet on the morning of the day your class meets so that it is complete the day before your next meeting. Use a pencil (not red) to fill out your Fact Sheet.

Most women in the program will be eating 1,200 calories each day. Men will usually eat 1,500. Expectant and nursing mothers should check with their doctors and team leaders. When your allotment is decided, record that number in the Daily Calories blank at the top of the Fact Sheet.

Next, refer to the First Place "Live-It" Plan in Appendix B to find the number of exchanges of each type of food you are allowed for each meal. Enter these numbers in the "Exchanges" boxes on the left side of the sheet.

Exchanges
1 Meat
1 Bread
1 Fruit
½ Milk
1 Fat

FIRST PLACE

Next, in the boxes under the day of the week, write first the amount and kind of food you ate adjacent to the square for that type of food. Chicken will be adjacent to the meat box, potatoes will be adjacent to the bread box, etc.

Next, determine how many exchanges the food counts and enter that number in the exchange box.

It is important that you do it in this order so you will write down all you ate before you try to calculate the amount of exchanges.

If you skip an exchange at any meal (even though it is recommended that you eat everything allowed at the time indicated or as a snack before the next meal), leave the box blank until the end of the day. At that time if you used that exchange or any part of that exchange at a different meal, put an asterisk in that box and show that food and exchange at the actual meal it was eaten. If at the end of the day you did not use the exchanges that you left blank, put a zero in that box. Please note that people who eat everything they are allowed, and have few zeros, are less likely to eat things they should not eat. Therefore they usually lose more than those who have more zeros. At the end of the day every box will have: an amount, an asterisk, or a zero. Always total the exchange at the bottom of the Fact Sheet each day

If you eat several items at one meal that constitute the same exchange, enter as shown below:

When you eat out and must estimate amounts, place a small "E" in the box with your exchange. Remember that it is always better to over-estimate than to under-estimate. Also remember that most foods eaten out have hidden fats in vegetables, soups, salads, as well as in meats.

Total all of your exchanges at the bottom of the Fact Sheet each day.

The back of the Fact Sheet is called the Awareness Record. This record will help you to see your weak areas and will enable your leader to assist you in seeing where you need to form new habits and break old ones.

When you are tempted to eat something you know you should not

Fact Sheet Information

be eating, or if you have had all of your fats and you want more, work through the Awareness Record.

If possible, do this *before* you eat the food and try to determine why you are having this problem. Try to resist eating it. Each time you are successful in resisting, it will make it easier the next time you try. However, if you give in and do not resist, it will make it easier the next time to give in again. Remember—*temptation—hesitation—participation*. Sometimes you do not have the opportunity to fill out the Awareness Record until *after* you have already lost the struggle and eaten the food. In this instance, be sure to go back and fill out the Awareness Record anyway.

There is a place on the back of the Fact Sheet next to the Awareness Record to record your faithfulness to the nine commitments. Fill them out daily.

Leave blank any commitment that you miss. Be consistent. Do not use any other markings or zeros. You will notice that you put the initial of the person whom you phoned. You are only required to make one phone call a week, but if you make others fill them in too. You are required to exercise three to five times a week. Leave blank any days you do not exercise.

Food for thought:

Proverbs 28:13—"He who conceals his transgressions will not prosper, but he who confesses and forsakes them will find compassion."

Proverbs 3:6—"In everything you do, put God first, and He will direct you and crown your efforts with success."

Be very careful that you are completely honest before the Lord on your Fact Sheets, not only on what you eat, but on the Awareness Record and Commitment Record. This is a commitment you made to Him and not to your leader. Your leader can only help you if he/she has all the facts.

You will turn your Fact Sheet in at each meeting. Before the next meeting, your leader will (with a red pen) go over your entire sheet

FIRST PLACE

circling errors, filling in boxes you failed to complete, and making comments and suggestions. Do not be alarmed by lots of red marks, as many of the comments will be positive remarks and praises for a good sheet. Red does not mean *bad*.

First Place Fact Sheet

Name _____ Date _____ thru _____ Daily Calories _____

Exchanges	Monday	Tuesday	Wednesday	Thursday	Friday	Saturday	Sunday
Morning — Meat, Bread, Fruit, Milk, Fat							
Midday — Meat, Bread, Veg., Fruit, Milk, Fat							
Evening — Meat, Bread, Veg., Fruit, Milk, Fat							
Daily Totals — Meat, Bread, Veg., Fruit, Milk, Fat, Water	___ Meat ___ Bread ___ Veg. ___ Fruit ___ Milk ___ Fat ___ Water	___ Meat ___ Bread ___ Veg. ___ Fruit ___ Milk ___ Fat ___ Water	___ Meat ___ Bread ___ Veg. ___ Fruit ___ Milk ___ Fat ___ Water	___ Meat ___ Bread ___ Veg. ___ Fruit ___ Milk ___ Fat ___ Water	___ Meat ___ Bread ___ Veg. ___ Fruit ___ Milk ___ Fat ___ Water	___ Meat ___ Bread ___ Veg. ___ Fruit ___ Milk ___ Fat ___ Water	___ Meat ___ Bread ___ Veg. ___ Fruit ___ Milk ___ Fat ___ Water

8

First Place Awareness Record

Commitments

Name _____
Loss _____ Gain _____
Dates _____ thru _____

Memory Verse: _____

Comments: _____

[1] **H: Degree of Hunger**
(0 = none, 3 = maximum)

[2] **BP: Body Position**
(1 = walking, 2 = standing,
3 = sitting, 4 = lying down)

	Prayer	Scripture Reading	Memory Verse	Bible Study	Phone Calls	Exercise	Distance	Time
Mon.								
Tues.								
Wed.								
Th.								
Fri.								
Sat.								
Sun.								

Day	Time	H[1]	BP[2]	Activity	Location	With	Feelings	Food

First Place Fact Sheet

Name Kay Smith Date June 9 thru June 15 Daily Calories 1200

	Exchanges		Monday		Tuesday		Wednesday		Thursday		Friday		Saturday		Sunday	
Morning	1	Meat	*		1	1 egg	1		*		*		1	1 egg	1	1 oz Canadian Bacon
	1	Bread	1	1/2 c. shredded wheat	1	2 slices diet whole wheat	1	1/2 bagel	1	1/2 c. oatmeal	1	1/2 bagel	2	1 flour tortilla 3 oz potato	1	2-4" pancakes
	1	Fruit	1	3 oz. banana	1	1 orange	1	1/2 grapefruit	1	1/2 c. orange	1	1 T. raisins 1/2 c. apple	1	1/2 c. fruit salad	1	1 1/4 c. strawberries
	1	Milk	1	8 oz. 1/2 %	*		1/2	4 oz. nonfat yogurt	1/2	4 oz. 1/2 %	1	8 oz. nonfat yogurt	*		1/2	4 oz. skim milk
	1	Fat	*		1/2	egg	*		*		*		1	1/2 = egg 1/2 = tortilla	1	=pancakes
Midday	2	Meat	2	c. tuna	2	2 oz. turkey	1	1 T. peanutbutter	2	1/2 c. cottage cheese	2	2 oz. lean ham	1	1 oz. cheese	2	2 oz. salmon
	2	Bread	2	1–6" pita bread	2	1 = 1 T c. pasta 1 = 1/2 c. spaghetti sauce	2	2 sl. whole wheat bread	1	5 melba toast	2	1/3 c. blackeyed peas 1/4 c. sweet potato	1	1=6 saltines	2	1= 2 1/2 T. cornmeal 1= whole grain roll
	1+	Veg.	1	1 c. tomatoes	1 1/2	1 = 1/2 c. mushrooms 1/2 = 1/2 c. tomatoes	1	1 c. carrots	2	2 c. raw cauliflower, broccoli, & carrots	2	1=1/2 c. beets 1=1/2 c. brussel sprouts	1	1/2 c. broccoli 1/2 c. carrots	1	1/2 c. eggplant
	1	Fruit	1	1 c. cantaloupe	1	15 grapes	1	1 pear	1	1/3 c. canned pineapple	*		1	3 oz banana	1	2 plums
	1/2	Milk	*		1	8 oz. nonfat yogurt	1	8 oz. 1/2 %	1/2	4 oz. nonfat yogurt	*		1/2	1 c. diet hot cocoa	1	8 oz. nonfat yogurt
	1	Fat	2	1 T diet mayo 1/8 avacado	1	2 T. Ranch	1	1 T. peanutbutter	1	1 tsp. salad dressing	1	1 T. diet marg.	1	1/2 = cheese 1/2 = 1 tsp. Ranch	1	1 tsp. oil
Evening	2	Meat	3	3 oz. lean beef	2	2 oz. fish	3	3 oz. chicken	3	3 oz. shrimp	3	2 oz lean beef 1 oz cheese	3	3 oz fish "E"	2	2 oz. chicken
	2	Bread	2	1/3 c. pinto beans 1–2" cornbread	2		2	1 corn tortilla 3 c. popcorn	2 1/2	2 = 2/3 c. rice 1/2 = cobbler	2	1 whole wheat bun	1	3 oz potato	2	1/3 c. brown rice 3/4 c. Fiber 1
	1+	Veg.	1	1/2 c. spinach	1	1/2 c. broccoli	1	1 c. tomato	2	1/2 c. cabbage 1/2 c. gr. beans	1/2	1/2 c. tomato	2	1 c. okra and tomatoes	2	1 c. tomatoes 1/2 c. carrots
	1	Fruit	1	3/4 c. peaches	1	1 1/4 c. strawberries	1	1 apple	1	3/4 c. blueberries	2	1 1/4 c watermelon 3 prunes	1	1 apple	1	1/3 cantoloupe
	1/2	Milk	1	1 pkg. alba	1	8 oz. 1/2 %	0		1/2	4 oz. nonfat yogurt	1	1 c. nonfat buttermilk	1/2	12 oz skim milk	1/2	4 oz. 1/2 %
	1	Fat	1	2" cornbread	1	1 T. diet marg.	1	1 T. diet marg.	1	1 = cobbler	2	1 T. diet mayo	1	1 T. diet marg.	1	20 sm peanuts

Daily Totals	Exchanges	Monday	Tuesday	Wednesday	Thursday	Friday	Saturday	Sunday
Meat	5	5	5	5	5	5	5	5
Bread	5	5	5	5	4 1/2	5	4	5
Veg.	2+	2	2 1/2	2	4	2 1/2	3	3
Fruit	3	3	3	3	3	3	3	3
Milk	2	2	2	1 1/2	1 1/2	2	2	2
Fat	3	3	2 1/2	2	2	3	3	3
Water	8	8+	8+	8+	8+	8	8+	8+

First Place Awareness Record
Commitments

Name: Kay Smith
Loss: −1 3/4   Gain: _____
Dates: June 9 thru June 15

Memory Verse: Set a guard O Lord over my mouth. Keep watch over the doors of my lips, Psalms 141:3

Comments: Please pray for Joe and me, we have an unspoken prayer request.

Kay call S. K. − 962-3713

[1] H: Degree of Hunger (0 = none, 3 = maximum)

[2] BP: Body Position (1 = walking, 2 = standing, 3 = sitting, 4 = lying down)

	Prayer	Scripture Reading	Memory Verse	Bible Study	Phone Calls	Exercise	Distance
Mon.	✓	PROVERBS 9 ACTS 9-10	✓ #7			walk	3 miles
Tues.	✓	PROVERBS 10 ACTS 11-12	✓ #1	✓ S.K.		walk	3 miles
Wed.	✓	PROVERBS 11 ACTS 13-14	✓ #2			walk	3 miles
Th.	✓	PROVERBS 12 ACTS 15-7	✓ #3			stationary bike	30 min.
Fri.	✓	PROVERBS 13 ACTS 18-19	✓ #4			walk	
Sat.	✓	PROVERBS 14 ACTS 20-21	✓ #5				
Sun.	✓	PROVERBS 15 ACTS 22-24	✓ #6				

Day	Time	H[1]	BP[2]	Activity	Location	With	Feelings	Food
Tues.	4:30 p.m.	3	2	cooking	kitchen	alone	tired/hungry	cheese
Thurs.	9:00 p.m.	0	3	reading	couch	Joe ♥	Good!	Everything! (made a legal strawberry milkshake)
Sat.	1:30 p.m.	1	2	shopping	mall	sister	tired/hungry	candy (made popcorn)
								(waited till I got to can- had apple)

Praise the LORD!

APPENDIX D

Breakfast—Why or Why Not?

Breakfast! Is skipping it really that bad for you? Is a good breakfast really all that important? The answer to both of these questions is yes!

Breakfast, the first meal of the day, usually occurs after at least an eight-hour fast. If you eat supper early in the evening, which is best, then the fast may be as long as twelve hours. A healthy body constantly maintains an appropriate blood sugar or glucose level so that you have an energy supply readily available for your daily needs. To work efficiently, you must maintain glucose levels. However, after a nightlong fast, your body will have to resupply the blood with glucose. If your body doesn't receive that nourishment in the form of a proper high-carbohydrate breakfast, then it must use the reserves it has stored in the liver. The constant withdrawal of your body's required amount of glucose each morning, in the form of glycogen, from your liver causes undue stress on the organ. Studies show that your mood and performance are affected by the foods you eat and especially by the lack of food, in this case. Certain mechanisms in the body, such as those which regulate appetite, fluid and electrolyte balance, and neurotransmitter levels in the brain, are adversely affected by missing the nutrition provided by a good breakfast.

FIRST PLACE

The most common excuse given for poor work performance is fatigue. The most apparent factors of fatigue are inadequate rest and excessive work, but nutritional deficiencies can contribute to fatigue just as much. Overall, poor eating habits diminish a person's abilities and can lead to exhaustion, apathy, poor concentration, and reduced strength.

UCLA's Center for Health Sciences conducted a study which monitored approximately seven thousand men and women. They found that the men who "rarely or sometimes" ate breakfast had 40 percent higher death rates than those men who ate breakfast "almost every day." They also found that the women who "rarely or sometimes" ate breakfast had 28 percent higher death rate than those women who ate breakfast "almost every day." These statistics are surprisingly high to many people. No one can predict for you if you will be one of those who suffer seriously from not eating a good breakfast, but we can warn that you place yourself in some risk if you don't. The University of Iowa did a long-term study that showed that better mental and physical performance among children and adults was directly associated with eating a nutritious breakfast. The subjects who ate breakfast were more productive and satisfied with their work performance during the late morning. Also, they had faster reaction times, which, in most instances, resulted in fewer accidents on the job.

One other risk is associated with skipping breakfast: You're likely to miss some very important nutrients, including vitamin C, thiamine (vitamin B), riboflavin (vitamin B2), iron, and calcium. These nutrients might be absent in the other meals of the day. Ninety-five percent of our food today is processed food and is low in essential nutrients. Going without breakfast only increases the chances that you won't consume all the essential nutrients.

Now that you know why it's bad to skip breakfast, what constitutes a nutritious breakfast? Bacon, fried eggs, buttered toast, and coffee may taste good, but they aren't the best foods to choose. They constitute a high-fat breakfast which gives you no advantage in starting your day. A good breakfast should average from 350 to 400 calories.

Breakfast—Why or Why Not?

These breakfast calories should be distributed as follows: 55 percent carbohydrates, 20 percent protein, and 25 percent fat. Some people believe in consuming a large breakfast, but actually, consuming more than 25 percent of your day's calories for breakfast reduces overall efficiency.

A large breakfast is not needed, but a balanced or properly distributed breakfast is essential.

Remember, a good breakfast is essential for good health. Don't take the chance of ruining your health by skipping breakfast!

BREAKFAST SUGGESTIONS

Each suggestion is one serving:

1. 1/4 cup cottage cheese
   1/2 apple, diced
   1 tablespoon raisins
   1/2 bagel

Exchanges: 1 meat, 1 fruit, and 1 bread

2. 2 slices whole-wheat diet bread (or 1 slice regular bread)
   1/4 cup cottage cheese
   1 grated apple, or fruit of choice
   1/2 teaspoon cinnamon
   1/2 package of artificial sweetener

Mix cottage cheese, apple, cinnamon, and sweetener. Put mixture on bread. Sprinkle with cinnamon and toast.

Exchanges: 1 meat, 1 bread, and 1 fruit

3. 8-ounce nonfat yogurt (sugar-free; fruit-type is fine)
   3 tablespoons grape nuts or cereal of choice

FIRST PLACE

    1 serving fruit, diced

Mix together and enjoy.

Exchanges: 1 bread, 1 milk, and 1 fruit

4. 1 egg, scrambled dry
   1 flour tortilla
   1 small red potato (1½ oz.)
   1 tablespoon onion (optional)

Microwave potato for 2 minutes and dice. Scramble egg. Spray pan with cooking spray and brown onion and diced potato. Place egg and potato mixture in a warm flour tortilla. Serve with pico de gallo or picante sauce.

Pico de gallo:
Chop 1 medium tomato, 2 tablespoons onion, 1 teaspoon hot pepper and cilantro to taste (approximately 2 tbsp.). Mix well.
Exchanges: 1 meat, 1 ½ breads and 1 fat
Pico de gallo; 1 cup = 1 vegetable
Pico de gallo is great on broiled fish, chicken, etc., and on salads if you like foods spicy.

5. Muffin (see Appendix F for recipes)
   8-ounce nonfat yogurt or 8-ounce skim milk
   1 serving fruit

Exchanges: muffin (according to exchanges in recipe section), 1 milk, and 1 fruit

APPENDIX E

Eating Out

1. Appetizers often can serve as the entree.
2. Request salad dressing on the side. Dipping your fork into the dressing will save a lot of fat.
3. Carry oil-free dressing with you.
4. Avoid all creamy salads. Starchy vegetables, creamy salads, and meat salads are loaded with sugar and fat.
5. Avoid marinated salads and pickled vegetables. They may contain sugar and fat.
6. Choose only fresh fruit. Many canned fruits contain sugar.
7. Select darkest greens available and add a variety of vegetables. Fresh spinach is an excellent salad base. Use spinach instead of lettuce, which provides very little nutrition.
8. Select lean meat entrees. Request that they be grilled dry without fat or butter.
9. Avoid all fried items.
10. Request that all sauces or gravy be served on the side. They are often full of sugar or fat.
11. Avoid casseroles and meat entrees in sauces. Chicken à la king, for example, averages 7 fats (35 grams) per serving.
12. Be creative—lemon juice and picante sauce are great on fish. You may want to carry packages of butter flavorings.
13. Your hand can serve as a measuring device when estimating meat servings. The average palm equals a 3-ounce serving of

meat ½-inch thick, the end section of your thumb a tablespoon, and the end section of your little finger a teaspoon.

14. Beware of "dieter specials." Specify nonfat and sugar-free when ordering! Many "diet" plates are full of fat and sugar.
15. Split the entree and order an extra salad. If alone, ask for the entree to be divided in half and packaged in a carryout before it comes to the table.
16. If you desire a substitution, ask for it, even when the menu states, "No substitutions." Restaurants usually are willing to accommodate special requests from regular customers.
17. If something comes with your order that you do not want, ask the waiter to leave it off the plate.
18. Request no butter or margarine on your bread.
19. Request baked potatoes and pasta dry. Mention that dry means no added fat.
20. Baked potatoes are great topped with steamed vegetables, picante sauce, jalapeños, lemon juice and pepper, ranch dressing, steak sauce, or cut-up meat. Be creative!
21. Request skim milk for coffee.
22. Fresh fruit is a good choice for dessert, or you might save a roll or bread to eat while others are having dessert.
23. Fast-food restaurants are now serving low-fat choices. Ask if chicken can be grilled dry. Choose wisely!
24. Enjoy the experience! Don't compromise your health and commitment!

APPENDIX F

Recipes

SALADS

Apple Salad Mold

Each serving amount: ½ cup
Exchanges: ½ fruit
Ingredients:
- 1 pkg. (3 oz.) sugar-free cherry Jell-O (or any flavor)
- 1 cup boiling water
- ½ cup apple juice
- ½ cup cold water
- 1 medium unpeeled apple, chopped (about 1½ cups)
- ½ cup chopped celery

Steps in Preparation:
1. Dissolve gelatin in boiling water.
2. Combine juice and cold water. Add to gelatin and stir.
3. Refrigerate until slightly thickened.
4. Add apple and celery; mix well.
5. Refrigerate until set.

Serves 5

FIRST PLACE

Diet 7-up Salad

Each serving amount: ½ cup
Exchanges: ¾ meat, ⅓ fruit, 1⅓ fat
Ingredients:
- 1½ cup crushed pineapple
- 1 cup hot water
- 1 small pkg. lime flavor sugar-free gelatin
- 1 pkg. (8 oz.) lite cream cheese
- 1 pkg. sugar substitute
- 1 tsp. vanilla
- 7 oz. diet lemon-lime soda

Steps in Preparation:
1. Drain pineapple, saving juice. Add enough hot water to juice to equal 1 cup. Bring to a boil.
2. Pour into blender and add gelatin and cheese. Blend on medium speed for 1 minute. Add pineapple and blend on low speed for 1 minute.
3. Pour into dish or mold and chill for 5 hours.

Serves 6

Pineapple Jell-O Salad

Each serving amount: ½ cup
Exchanges: ½ fruit
Ingredients:
- 1 can (20 oz.) crushed pineapple, drained
- 2 pkgs. (4-serving size) sugar-free Jell-O (any flavor)
- Fat-free Cool Whip

Steps in Preparation:
1. Make Jell-O per package directions.
2. Divide pineapple into 10 dessert dishes.
3. Pour Jell-O over pineapple.
4. Chill until set.
5. Top with Fat-free Cool Whip.

Serves 10.

Pineapple Jell-O Salad

Same as above but add 1 cup grated carrots to pineapple. Serve on a bed of lettuce.
Serves 10

Pasta Salad

Each serving amount: 1 cup
Exchanges: 2 breads, 1/2 vegetable
Ingredients:
- 3 quarts water
- 4 chicken bouillon cubes
- 1 Tbs. seasoned salt
- 16 oz. pkg. penne rigate pasta
- 1 green bell pepper, sliced thin
- 1 red bell pepper, sliced thin
- 1 yellow bell pepper, sliced thin
- 1 8 oz. pkg. fresh mushrooms, sliced
- 12 black olives, sliced thin
- 1 bunch green onion tops, chopped
- Fat-free oil dressing (recipe below)

Steps in Preparation:
1. Add bouillon cubes and seasoned salt to water. Bring to boil.
2. Add pasta. Boil until tender. Drain
3. Add green bell pepper, red bell pepper, yellow bell pepper, mushrooms, olives, and green onion tops.
4. Pour dressing over pasta and mix well. Refrigerate until ready to serve.

Variations:
- Top with 2 oz. grilled chicken - 2 meats
- Top with 2 oz. shrimp - 1 meat
- Top with 2 oz. tuna - 1 meat

Serves 12

FIRST PLACE

Fat-Free Oil Dressing

Exchanges: free
Ingredients:
- 8 oz. fat-free Italian dressing
- 2 Tbs. balsamic vinegar
- 1½ tsp. dried basil leaves

Steps in Preparation:
1. Mix all ingredients.
2. Refrigerate until ready to serve. *Will last indefinitely in the refrigerator.

Raspberry Vinaigrette

Each serving amount: 2 tablespoons
Exchanges: Free
Ingredients:
- ½ cup rice vinegar
- ⅓ cup seedless raspberry all-fruit jelly
- 2 Tbs. applesauce
- 2 Tbs. chopped pecans

Steps in Preparation:
1. Combine all ingredients.
2. Blend well.
3. Refrigerate until ready to serve.

Serves 8

Recipes

MAIN DISHES

Stay-Slim Lasagna

Each serving amount: $1/6$ of lasagna pan
Exchanges: 3 meat, 1 bread, $1\frac{1}{2}$ vegetable, $1/2$ fat
Ingredients:
- $1/2$ lb. ground turkey or beef
- $1/4$ cup chopped onion
- 1 clove garlic, finely chopped
- $1/2$ tsp. Italian dressing
- $1/2$ tsp. basil
- 1 Tbs. dried parsley
- $1/4$ tsp. crushed red pepper (optional)
- salt and pepper to taste
- 6 lasagna noodles
- 1 (6 oz.) can tomato paste + 1 can water
- 1 cup sliced fresh mushrooms or 4 oz. can mushrooms, drained
- 10 oz. fresh or frozen spinach leaves, chopped
- 2 Tbs. finely chopped onion
- 6 oz. low-fat ricotta cheese
- $1/2$ clove garlic, finely chopped
- 6 oz. mozzarella cheese shredded (reserve 3 oz. for top)

Steps in Preparation:
1. Sauté beef, onion, garlic. Add seasonings, tomato paste, and water. Simmer about 10 minutes. Stir in mushrooms.
2. Steam fresh spinach, onion, and garlic, stirring occasionally, until spinach is wilted. Mash out excess liquid, using wire strainer. (For frozen spinach, thaw and mash out excess water.) Add $1/4$ tsp. black pepper if desired. Stir until well blended. Mix in ricotta and 3 oz. of mozzarella.
3. Boil 6 lasagna noodles until tender; drain.
4. In 9x9 square or 7x11 casserole dish layer, 3 noodles; $1/2$ meat mixture; entire spinach/cheese layer; 3 noodles; remaining meat mixture.

FIRST PLACE

5. Bake at 350 degrees for 30 minutes. Top with 3 oz. mozzarella. Serves 6

Cheddar Cheese Soup

Each serving amount: 10 ounces
Exchanges: $1/2$ lean meat, $1/4$ bread, $1/2$ milk, $1 1/2$ fat
Ingredients:
- $1/2$ cup carrots, finely chopped
- 1 cup celery, finely chopped
- 1 cup green onions, finely chopped
- 2 cups water
- 1 medium white onion, chopped
- 2 Tbs. diet margarine
- 1 cup flour
- 4 cups skim or $1/2$ percent milk
- 4 cups chicken broth
- 1 (15 oz.) jar Cheez Whiz, light
- salt and pepper to taste
- $1/4$ tsp. cayenne pepper
- 1 Tbs. prepared mustard

Steps in Preparation:
1. Boil carrots, celery, and green onions in water 5 minutes.
2. Sauté white onion in butter. Add flour and blend well.
3. Boil milk and chicken broth. Stir briskly into white onion mixture with a wire whisk. Add Cheez Whiz, salt, pepper, and cayenne. Stir in mustard and the boiled vegetables, including the water in which they were cooked. Bring to a boil and serve immediately.
4. We do not recommend chopping these ingredients in a food processor.

Serves 16

Recipes

White Bean Soup

Each serving amount: ½ cup of beans plus ½ cup liquid to equal 1 cup
Exchanges: 1 bread
Ingredients:
- 1 pound package navy beans or great northern beans
- 4 chicken bouillon cubes
- seasoned salt, as desired
- 4 cloves garlic, chopped
- 1 onion, chopped finely
- 1 cup carrots, chopped
- 1 cup celery, chopped
- 1 cup corn, frozen

Steps in Preparation:
1. Cover navy beans with 3 inches of water. Add bouillon cubes, garlic, seasoned salt, and onion. Boil gently until almost done, approximately 1½ hours.
2. Add carrots and celery and cook until tender.
3. Add corn and cook for another 8 minutes.

Note: If extra water is needed while beans are cooking, bring water to boil before adding to beans.
Serves 8

French Bread Vegetable Pizza

Each serving amount: one slice
Exchanges (each slice): 2 meats, 2 breads, ½ vegetable, 1 fat
Ingredients:
- 2 oz. piece french bread
- pizza sauce (recipe follows)
- 2 oz. mozzarella cheese
- choice of vegetable, sliced thinly (onions, mushrooms, bell pepper, zucchini squash)

FIRST PLACE

Steps in Preparation:
1. Top bread with thin layer of pizza sauce (approximately $1\frac{1}{2}$ Tbs.) and mozzarella cheese.
2. Cover with choice of vegetables.
3. Bake at 375 degrees until cheese melts, approximately 15 minutes.

Variations:
1. Use 2 oz. bagel in place of French bread.
2. Use 2 oz. English muffin in place of French bread.

Serves 1

Pizza Sauce

Ingredients:
- $1\frac{1}{2}$ cups water
- 1 Tbs. basil
- $\frac{1}{2}$ Tbs. oregano
- 1 can (12 oz.) tomato sauce
- 1 can (6 oz.) tomato paste

Steps in Preparation:
1. Combine $1\frac{1}{2}$ cups water, basil, and oregano and bring to boil. Let steep for 3–5 minutes.
2. Add tomato sauce and tomato paste. Simmer until desired thickness is obtained.

Serves 12

Pasta Sauce

Each serving amount: 6 ounces
Exchanges: 1 vegetable, $\frac{1}{3}$ bread

Ingredients:
- 2 cups water
- 4 Tbs. basil
- 2 Tbs. oregano

Recipes

    8 chicken bouillon cubes
    2 cans crushed tomatoes (14½ oz. size cans)
    1 can (6 oz.) tomato paste
    1½ cups onion, finely chopped
    8–10 cloves garlic, crushed
    ½ tsp. cayenne pepper

Steps in Preparation:
1. Combine 2 cups of water, basil, oregano, and bouillon cubes. Bring to a boil. Steep 3–5 minutes. Pour through tea strainer and discard basil, etc. Save water.
2. Add tomatoes, tomato paste, onion, garlic, and pepper to water.
3. Simmer 45 minutes or until thick.

Serves 6

Note: Bouillon should provide enough salt.

Variations:
1. Any pasta can be used; spaghetti, linguini, etc. Exchange: ½ cup = 1 bread
2. Add 2 ounces sliced grilled chicken on top of sauce. Exchange: 2 meats
3. Add ½ cup steamed mixed vegetables. Exchange: 1 vegetable

Johnny's Cajun Meatloaf

Each serving amount: 1/10 of loaf
Exchanges: 1 slice = 3 meats, ½ bread
Ingredients:
    2 pounds ground round
    ¾ cup finely chopped onions
    ½ cup finely chopped celery
    ½ cup finely chopped green bell pepper
    ¼ cup finely chopped green onion tops
    2 tsp. minced garlic
    3 Tbs. *Pickapeppa sauce
    1 Tbs. Worcestershire sauce

FIRST PLACE

½ cup catsup
½ cup skim milk
3 egg whites, lightly beaten
1 cup Progresso plain dry bread crumbs
1 Tbs. salt
½ tsp. cayenne pepper
1 tsp. black pepper

Steps in Preparation:
1. Mix all ingredients together, shape into loaf and place in ungreased pan.
2. Bake uncovered 25 minutes at 350 degrees.
3. Make a sauce of 3 oz. catsup and 1 Tbs. *Pickapeppa sauce.
4. Remove meatloaf from oven and spread sauce on top.
5. Heat to 400 degrees and cook 30 minutes more.

*If Pickapeppa sauce is not available in your area, use your favorite steak sauce as a substitution.

Serves 10

Superb Chili and Beans

Each serving amount: 1 cup
Exchanges: 2 meats, 1 bread
Ingredients:

3 pounds ground round or ground sirloin
1 cup chopped onions
8 oz. tomato sauce
2 cups water
3½ Tbs. (heaping) chili powder
1 tsp. oregano
1 tsp. (heaping) cumin
6 garlic cloves chopped
1 Tbs. (heaping) salt
1 tsp. paprika

# Recipes

Steps in Preparation:
1. Brown ground meat with 1 cup chopped onions until meat is gray in color. Drain all excess liquid from pan.
2. Add remaining ingredients.
3. Simmer one hour and fifteen minutes.
   *use Teflon pot, if possible

At the same time, cook pinto beans:

Ingredients:
- 1 lb. pinto beans, rinsed
- 5 quarts water
- 1 Tbs. seasoned salt
- 1 Tbs. (heaping) chili powder
- 1 tsp. cumin
- 1 tsp. paprika

Steps in Preparation:
1. Put all ingredients in 1½ gallon pot. Boil gently 1½ hours and taste for seasoning.
2. Boil gently an additional 1½ hours.
3. Add to cooked chili and heat on LOW for 30 minutes, stirring often.

Serves 20

Taco Soup

Each serving amount: 1½ cups
Exchanges: 1⅓ meats, 1½ breads, ¾ vegetable

Ingredients:
- 16 oz. extra lean ground round (measurement is after meat has been browned)
- 1 cup onion, chopped
- 2½ cups carrots, sliced
- 3 cups pinto beans (measurement is after beans have been thoroughly rinsed and drained)
- 2 cups corn (measurement is after corn has been drained)

FIRST PLACE

   3 cups red potatoes, peeled and diced
   4 beef bouillon cubes
   1 pkg. mild taco seasoning
   1 pkg. ranch dressing mix
   1¼ cups Rotel Tomatoes and Chilies
   8 cups water (or use 10 cups of water for more broth)

Steps in Preparation:
1. Lightly brown ground round in large skillet. Drain meat in colander and rinse with very hot water.
2. Lightly sauté onions in a little water with the 4 bouillon cubes.
3. Combine onions and meat with remaining ingredients. Bring to boil and simmer 20–30 minutes.

Serve with Baked Tostitos, fat-free saltine crackers, or low-fat cornbread.

Serves 10

Variations:
1. Substitute chicken breast or extra lean ground turkey for the ground round. If chicken is substituted, use chicken bouillon cubes instead of beef.
2. Substitute stewed tomatoes for Rotel Tomatoes and Chilies.
3. Substitute hominy for corn.
4. Cook dried pinto beans from scratch and use 3 cups of beans in recipe.
5. Add jalapeño peppers for a hotter and spicier taste.

Vegetarian Quesadillas

Each serving amount: 1 tortilla
Exchanges: 2 meats, 2 breads, 1 vegetable, 1 fat
Ingredients:
   6 large flour tortillas
   1½ cups onion, sliced thin
   1½ cups mushrooms, sliced thin
   1½ cups carrots, sliced thin

Recipes

 1½ cups broccoli, chopped
 12 oz. mozzarella cheese

Steps in Preparation:
1. Sauté vegetables in skillet sprayed with non-stick cooking spray until done, yet crisp.
2. Heat griddle.
3. Place tortilla on hot griddle and sprinkle with 2 oz. cheese.
4. When cheese begins to melt, cover ½ of tortilla with ½ cup of vegetables.
5. Fold over tortilla and grill until hot.
6. Slice in three triangle sections.
7. Serve with Picante sauce or salsa.

Variation:
Add 1 oz. chopped chicken breast to quesadilla. Exchange - 1 meat.
Serves 6

Mega Chicken Vegetable Soup

Each serving amount: 8 oz.
Exchanges: ¾ meat, 1 bread, 1½ vegetables
Ingredients:
 3 quarts water
 8 oz. tomato sauce
 10 chicken bouillon cubes
 4 cups potatoes, cubed
 3 cups carrots, sliced ½-inch thick
 3 cups zucchini squash
 2 cups onion, chopped coarse
 2 cups corn, fresh or frozen
 3 cups green beans, fresh or frozen
 1 lb. skinless, boneless chicken breasts

Steps in Preparation:
1. Boil chicken breasts in 3 quarts of water. Remove breasts and save broth.

FIRST PLACE

2. Add remaining ingredients to broth and boil 45 minutes or until vegetables are firm, yet done.
3. Cut chicken breasts into bite-size pieces and add to soup.

Serves 12

Chicken Supreme

Serving amount: 1 chicken breast
Exchanges: 3 meats, 1/2 bread
Ingredients:
    5 3 oz. chicken breasts
    1 cup bread crumbs
    1 tsp. salt
    1/4 tsp. black pepper
    1 cup grated parmesan cheese
    2 Tbs. parsley
    1 clove garlic, crushed
    1/4 oz. slivered almonds (save a few for topping)
    3 egg whites

Steps in Preparation:
1. Combine bread crumbs, parmesan cheese, salt, pepper, parsley, garlic, and almonds.
2. Dip chicken in egg whites, and then roll in bread crumb mixture. Arrange in 9x13 baking dish, and sprinkle with a few slivered almonds.
3. Bake at 350 degrees for 30 minutes.

Serves 6

Pinto Beans à la Juan

Each serving amount: 1/2 cup
Exchanges: 1 bread, 1 vegetable
Ingredients:
    2 lbs. pinto beans, rinsed

Recipes

    10 quarts water
    6 whole garlic cloves (discard after 2 hours cooking)
    1 large onion, chopped medium coarse
    1 heaping Tbs. chili powder
    1 heaping Tbs. Tony's Creole Seasoning
    1 heaping Tbs. Goya Adobo
    1 heaping Tbs. salt

Steps in Preparation:
1. Mix all ingredients.
2. In 3 gallon pot, boil gently 1½ hours and taste for seasoning.
3. Cook 5 hours total on low rolling boil.

For cilantro beans:
When beans are tender, add:
    2 medium bell peppers, chopped medium coarse
    4 firm tomatoes, chopped medium coarse
    1 large yellow onion, chopped coarse
    1 bunch cilantro, rinsed and tied (discard cilantro after beans are done)

Cornbread Dressing

Each serving amount: ½ cup
Exchanges: 1½ breads, ½ fat
Ingredients:
    1 8 oz. pkg. herb-seasoned cornbread stuffing mix
    2 6 oz. pkg. cornbread mix
    2 whole eggs
    1⅓ cups skim milk
    1½ cups onion, chopped
    1½ cups celery, chopped
    10 chicken bouillon cubes
    10 cups water
    1 Tbs. poultry seasoning
    4 egg whites

FIRST PLACE

Steps in Preparation:
1. Make cornbread according to package directions, using the 2 whole eggs and skim milk.
2. Boil celery and onion in the water with the bouillon cubes over low heat for 3–5 minutes.
3. Crumble cooked cornbread and combine with stuffing mix.
4. Pour boiled mixture over bread mixture.
5. After mixture has cooled, stir in beaten egg whites.
6. Bake at 375 degrees for 45 minutes.

Serves 16

Gravy for Cornbread Dressing

Each serving amount: 1/4 cup
Exchanges: Free
Ingredients:
- 3/4 quart water
- 4 chicken bouillon cubes
- 2 Tbs. flour
- salt and pepper to taste

Steps in Preparation:
1. In a pan, bring water to boil. Add bouillon cubes.
2. In a pint jar with lid, combine 3/4 cup of the bouillon water with flour.
3. Shake well.
4. Pour this mixture into remaining water, a little at a time to prevent lumping.
5. Cook over low heat, stirring frequently, until gravy consistency.
6. May add more flour and water if needed.

Serves 16

Recipes

BREADS

Very Berry Blueberry Muffins

Each serving amount: 1 muffin
Exchanges: $\frac{1}{2}$ bread, $\frac{1}{2}$ fruit
Ingredients:
- 1 cup mashed banana
- 2 egg whites or 1 jumbo egg
- $\frac{1}{2}$ cup unsweetened pineapple juice concentrate (Minute Maid)
- $\frac{1}{4}$ cup vanilla yogurt
- 1 Tbs. water
- 2 cups low-fat Pioneer Baking Mix (or low-fat Bisquick mix)
- 1 cup fresh or frozen blueberries, left to thaw in a strainer
- 2 tsp. baking soda
- $\frac{1}{8}$ tsp. salt
- 1 pkg. of sugar substitute

Steps in Preparation:
1. Preheat oven to 350 degrees.
2. Prepare 18 standard-sized cups with paper liners.
3. In a large bowl, stir together banana, egg, oil, pineapple concentrate, and water. Add flour and mix. Gently stir in blueberries. Stir in baking soda quickly and then mix (28 to 30 strokes).
4. Spoon batter into prepared muffin cups. Bake about 20 minutes or until a toothpick inserted in the center of one muffin comes out clean.
5. Remove muffins from pan immediately and sprinkle with one package of Equal, if desired.
6. Cool on a wire rack.
7. Serve warm or cool completely and store in an airtight container in the refrigerator or freezer.

Serves 18

FIRST PLACE

Tropical Muffins

Each serving amount: 1 muffin
Exchanges: 1 bread, 1 fat
Ingredients:
- 1¾ cup all-purpose flour
- sugar substitute to equal ¾ cup sugar
- 2 tsp. baking powder
- ¼ tsp. baking soda
- ½ tsp. salt
- ¼ cup unsweetened grated coconut
- 3 medium-size ripe bananas, mashed
- ⅓ cup reduced-calorie margarine, melted
- 1 egg, beaten
- 1 tsp. grated orange rind
- ⅓ cup unsweetened orange juice
- vegetable cooking spray

Steps in Preparation:
1. Sift together flour, sugar substitute, baking powder, soda, and salt in a large bowl; stir in coconut, and make a well in center of mixture.
2. Combine bananas, margarine, egg, orange rind, and juice; add to dry ingredients, stirring just until dry ingredients are moistened.
3. Spoon batter into muffin pans coated with cooking spray, filling two-thirds full. Bake at 375 degrees for 25 to 30 minutes or until lightly browned.

Helpful Hint:
Use all vegetable margarine or oil instead of butter, lard, or solid shortening when baking. Also, remember that any fat added to bread after baking or to cereals after cooking must be calculated into your meal plan in order to control calories.
Serves 12

Recipes

DESSERTS

Blue Ribbon Frozen Snicker Dessert

Each serving amount: ⅛ of dessert
Exchanges: ½ meat, 1 bread, ½ fat
Ingredients:
- 12 oz. frozen vanilla yogurt or ice cream (fat-free and sugar-free)
- 1 cup Fat-free Cool Whip
- 3 Tbs. chunky peanut butter
- 1 pkg. (4 serving size) instant sugar-free chocolate pudding, dry
- 3 graham cracker squares (½ cup crumbs)

Steps in Preparation:
1. Crush the graham cracker squares into fine crumbs and place in an 8 x 8 baking dish.
2. Mix all other ingredients together.
3. Pour into dish, being careful not to disturb crumbs.
4. Freeze until firm.
5. To serve, remove from freezer 10 minutes before serving. Cut into 8 equal portions.

Serves 8

Banana Berry Cream Pie

Each serving amount: ⅛ of pie
Exchanges: ½ meat, 1 bread, ½ fruit, ½ fat
Ingredients:
- 4 oz. fat-free cream cheese
- 1 pkg. (4 serving size) sugar-free instant vanilla pudding
- 1 cup skim milk
- 4 oz. Fat-free Cool Whip
- 2 Tbs. all-fruit jelly (whatever flavor goes best with berries)
- 1 medium banana
- 1 cup berries (sliced strawberries, blueberries, raspberries, or mixed)

FIRST PLACE

    1 reduced-fat graham cracker crust

Steps in Preparation:
1. Slice banana and layer in bottom of pie shell.
2. Arrange berries on top of bananas.
3. Beat cream cheese and jelly with mixer until smooth. Fold in Cool Whip.
4. In separate bowl, mix milk and pudding mix until smooth (will be thick).
5. Pour pudding over fruit and spread evenly.
6. Top with cream cheese mixture. Chill a few hours for best results.

Serves 8

First Place Banana Pudding

Each serving amount: 1/6 of pudding
Exchanges: 1/2 bread, 1 fruit, 1/2 milk
Ingredients:
    3/4 cup graham cracker crumbs
    1 small box sugar-free Jell-O banana pudding + 2 cups 1/2 percent milk
    3 bananas
    1 cup Fat-free Cool Whip

Steps in Preparation:
1. Sprinkle graham cracker crumbs on bottom of pan.
2. Slice bananas and layer on top of graham cracker crumbs.
3. Prepare pudding as directed and pour over bananas.
4. Spread Fat-free Cool Whip on top.
5. Refrigerate until ready to serve.

Serves 6

Recipes

Chocolate Eclair Dessert

Each serving amount: 1 portion
Exchanges: 1 bread, ¼ milk
Ingredients:
- 24 low-fat graham crackers (about 1 box)
- 2 small sugar-free instant vanilla pudding
- 3 cups skim milk
- 1 pkg. (12 oz.) Fat-free Cool Whip
- 1 small sugar-free instant chocolate pudding

Steps in Preparation:
1. Place 8 crackers in bottom of 13 x 9 pan.
2. Mix vanilla pudding and milk well; let sit 2 minutes.
3. Gently fold in Fat-free Cool Whip.
4. Pour half on graham crackers.
5. Top with another 8 crackers.
6. Pour remaining pudding over crackers.
7. Top with last 8 crackers.
8. Mix the small instant chocolate pudding with 1½ cups skim milk. Let sit 2 minutes. Spread over graham crackers.
9. Let sit 6 hours or overnight in refrigerator to soften crackers.
10. Strawberries may be served on top for garnish.

Serves 18

Lemon Icebox Dessert

Each serving amount: ⅛ of dessert
Exchanges: 1 bread, ¼ milk
Ingredients:
- 2 cups skim milk
- ½ tub Crystal Light lemonade mix, dry
- 1 large box vanilla sugar-free instant pudding, dry
- 1 pkg. (8 oz.) Fat-free Cool Whip
- 6 graham cracker squares (3-inch)

FIRST PLACE

Steps in Preparation:
1. Layer graham crackers in the bottom of an 8 x 8 baking dish.
2. In a mixing bowl, stir pudding and lemonade powder together, then add milk and mix on low speed of hand mixer.
3. Add three-fourths of the Fat-free Cool Whip.
4. Pour mixture on graham crackers and top with remaining Fat-free Cool Whip.
5. Refrigerate until ready to serve.

Serves 8

Banana Split Dessert

Each serving amount: 1 portion
Exchanges: 1 bread, 1/4 milk, 1/2 fruit
Ingredients:
    24 low-fat graham crackers (about 1 box)
    2 small sugar-free instant banana pudding
    3 cups skim milk + 1 1/2 cups skim milk
    1 pkg. (10 oz.) Fat-free Cool Whip (thawed)
    1 small sugar-free instant chocolate pudding
    1 can (16 oz.) crushed pineapple (only need half) drained
    2 bananas
    chopped pecans (very few)

Steps in Preparation:
1. Place 8 crackers in bottom of 13 x 9 cake pan.
2. Mix banana pudding and 3 cups milk well; let sit 2 minutes.
3. Stir in drained pineapple.
4. Gently fold in Fat-free Cool Whip.
5. Pour half over graham crackers.
6. Slice bananas and place on top of pudding.
7. Top with another 8 crackers.
8. Pour remaining pudding with pineapples over crackers.
9. Top with sliced strawberries.
10. Top with last 8 crackers.

Recipes

11. Mix the chocolate pudding with 1½ cups milk; let sit 2 minutes.
12. Spread over graham crackers.
13. Let sit 6 hours or overnight in refrigerator to soften crackers. Cut into 18 pieces.
14. Sprinkle with pecans.

Serves 18

Strawberry Surprise

Each serving amount: ½ cup
Exchanges: ¼ bread, ½ milk, ½ fruit
Ingredients:
- 1 carton (32 oz.) Vanilla-flavored Dannon Light Yogurt (or other low-calorie/low-fat brand)
- 4 cartons (8 oz. each) Banana Cream Pie-flavored Dannon Light Yogurt
- 1 carton (8 oz.) Fat-free Cool Whip
- 5 cups strawberries
- 2 bananas (about 9 in. each)
- 1 small pkg. Strawberry Banana-flavored Sugar-free Jell-O (dry powder)
- 2 cups "Honey Bunches of Oats" cereal (crushed) (Grapenuts or other cereals could be used, but check serving sizes)

Steps in Preparation:
1. Blend the yogurt and Fat-free Cool Whip together in a large bowl. Stir in the Jell-O powder and blend well. Best when refrigerated several hours, then stirred again before serving, but if desired it can be served immediately.
2. Slice strawberries and bananas, then divide evenly into serving bowls.
3. Dividing evenly, spoon yogurt mixture over fruit.
4. Crush the cereal, sprinkle 1 tablespoon over each serving.

FIRST PLACE

Variations: Other flavors of low-calorie dairy yogurt and sugar-free Jell-O can be used, as well as, other fruits of choice. If desired, the topping could be omitted, eliminating the bread count.
Serves 16
Individual servings can be made by using:
- 8 oz. Dannon Light Yogurt (flavor of choice)
- 2 Tbs. Fat-free Cool Whip
- ½ tsp. sugar-free Jell-O powder
- ¼ banana
- ½ cup strawberries
- 1 Tbs. cereal

Exchanges for individual serving: ¼ bread, 1 milk, 1 fruit

Fruit Crisp

Each serving amount: ⅙ of recipe
Exchanges: 1 fruit
Ingredients:
- 1 Tbs. sugar
- ¼ tsp. cinnamon
- 4 cups peeled, sliced apples, pears or peaches

Steps in Preparation:
1. Combine sugar and cinnamon.
2. Place fruit in a 9-inch pie plate.
3. Sprinkle mixture over fruit. Toss gently to coat.
4. Cover and bake at 375 degrees for 25 minutes.

Topping
Ingredients:
- ¼ cup quick-cooking rolled oats
- 1 Tbs. brown sugar
- 2½ Tbs. flour
- 1 Tbs. diet margarine (melted)
- ¼ tsp. cinnamon

Steps in Preparation:
1. Mix all topping ingredients. Sprinkle over partially cooked fruit.
2. Return to oven and bake, uncovered 15–20 minutes or until fruit is tender.

Serves 6

Blue Ribbon Brownies

Each serving amount: 3 brownies
Exchanges: 1 bread, $1/4$ milk, $1/2$ fat
Ingredients:
- 1½ cups non-fat Pioneer Baking Mix
- 1 carton (8 oz.) Dannon Lite Creme Caramel Yogurt
- 4 Tbs. cocoa
- 4 pkgs. Sweet-n-Low
- 1 tsp. vanilla
- 1 egg (jumbo)
- ¼ cup canned evaporated skim milk
- 5 pecans (chopped)
- 2 pkgs. Equal

Steps in Preparation:
1. Combine all ingredients except pecans.
2. Pour into 9 x 13 baking pan sprayed with Pam.
3. Sprinkle pecans on top of batter and bake at 350 degrees for 15 minutes.
4. Cool 10 minutes, then sprinkle 2 packages of Equal on top. Cut into 24 squares.

Serves 8

To make Brownie Truffle:
Each serving amount: $1/12$ of truffle
Exchanges: ¾ milk, 1 bread, 1 fat
Ingredients:
- Blue Ribbon Brownies
- 1 large box of sugar-free vanilla pudding

FIRST PLACE

    1 large box of sugar-free chocolate pudding
    1 pkg. Cool Whip Lite
    nuts

Steps for Preparation:
1. Bake brownies using Blue Ribbon Brownie recipe.
2. Prepare large box of sugar-free vanilla pudding and a large box of sugar-free chocolate pudding according to box instructions.
3. After the brownies have cooled, break up half of them in the bottom of a deep bowl. Next, layer half of the chocolate pudding, half of the vanilla pudding and repeat layers.
4. Top with Fat-free Cool Whip and a few nuts.

Serves 12

Three-Layer Apple Raisin Pie

Each serving amount: $1/8$ of pie
Exchanges: $1\frac{1}{4}$ bread, 1 fruit, $\frac{1}{2}$ milk, $1\frac{1}{2}$ fat
Ingredients:
    1 pkg. dried apples
    $\frac{1}{2}$ cup raisins
    1 tsp. cinnamon
    1 Tbs. cornstarch
    1 large package sugar-free vanilla pudding
    1 pkg. sugar-free whipped topping prepared with $\frac{1}{2}$ cup milk instead of water
    4 packets sugar substitutes (add to cooked, cooled apples)

Steps in Preparation:
1. Add three cups water to the dried apples, soak a few minutes if time permits.
2. Cook at low heat for 30 minutes. Add raisins and cinnamon and cook another 15 minutes.
3. Dissolve cornstarch with a small amount of water and add to boiling apples. Cook 5 minutes and set aside to cool. After apples have cooled, add to a cooked, cooled pie crust.

4. Mix pudding according to directions. Pour pudding over the apple filling and place in the refrigerator while preparing the low-calorie whipping topping. Add the topping and refrigerate.

Serves 8

Creamy Pumpkin Soufflé

Each serving amount: ½ cup
Exchanges: ½ bread
Ingredients:
- 1 large package vanilla sugar-free instant pudding
- 1 can (16 oz.) pumpkin
- 1 cup milk (½ percent)
- ½ tsp. nutmeg
- ½ teaspoon ginger
- ½ teaspoon cinnamon
- 1 cup Fat-free Cool Whip

Steps in Preparation:
1. Combine pudding and milk; add pumpkin and spices in a bowl. Fold in Fat-free Cool Whip.
2. Pour into pudding cups, chill and serve

Serves 8

Variation:
Serve in graham cracker pie crust. (Exchanges: 1½ bread, 1 fat)

Apple Cobbler

Each serving amount: ⅛ of cobbler
Exchanges: 1½ fruits, ½ bread, ¼ fat
Ingredients for filling:
- 6 oz. can frozen apple juice concentrate (unsweetened and undiluted)
- 2 Tbs. cornstarch
- 1 Tbs. reduced fat margarine

FIRST PLACE

    1 tsp. cinnamon
    1 tsp. vanilla extract
    6 medium apples (peeled, cored and sliced)

Steps in Preparation of filling:
1. Combine apple juice and cornstarch.
2. Cook over medium heat until thick and bubbly.
3. Stir in margarine, cinnamon, and vanilla.
4. Add apples and toss.
5. Pour into 9-inch pie pan.
6. Make topping recipe as follows.

Ingredients for Topping:
    ½ cup flour
    ⅛ tsp. salt
    ⅛ tsp. nutmeg
    2 Tbs. reduced fat margarine

Steps in Preparation of Topping:
1. Mix all ingredients to form crumble topping.
2. Sprinkle over apple mixture.
3. Bake cobbler at 350 degrees for 30 minutes. Excellent served warm.

Serves 8

APPENDIX G

Exercise Basics and Exercise Log

BURNING CALORIES IS KEY TO EXERCISE BENEFITS

Burning calories in moderate exercise rather than engaging in activity that requires "superhuman effort" produces a wide range of health benefits, says Dr. William Haskell, associate professor of medicine and associate doctor for Stanford University's Center for Research in Disease Prevention.

He points out that although most exercise regimens target particular heart rates or rates of oxygen consumption as goals, the key stimulus that promotes beneficial physiological changes in the body is an increase in energy production, which means burning calories.

His recommended allowance of exercise for good health calls for the expenditure of 1.8 calories for each pound of body weight at least every other day. For example, if you weigh 160 pounds, your calorie expenditure would be 288. This, says Dr. Haskell, is the minimal energy use needed to derive physiological benefits from exercise, based on numerous epidemiological and physiological studies.

A calorie, incidentally, is a unit of heat, defined as the amount of heat needed to change the temperature of one kilogram of water from 14.5 degrees Celsius to 15.5 degrees Celsius.

Dr. Haskell's minimal exercise allowance for the average 165-pound man translates into approximately thirty to forty minutes of rigorous exercise every other day or forty-five to sixty minutes of moderate exercise such as brisk walking. "Intensity and duration are always a trade-off in exercise," he notes.

Significant health benefits can be achieved from low-intensity exercise regimens focused on burning calories, says Dr. Haskell. Only slightly more benefits come from increasing the activity of an already active person, he adds.

In adapting to the stress of exercise, the body undergoes beneficial physiological changes that occur during and immediately after exercise, which leads to more efficient metabolism and reduced risk of developing coronary artery disease, as well as psychological benefits, according to Dr. Haskell.

Additional benefits of regular activity are an increased sensitivity to insulin, decreased levels of triglycerides in the blood, improved blood-clotting mechanisms, and an increased ratio of high-density lipoprotein (HDL)—good in terms of cholesterol—to low-density lipoprotein (LDL), the bad cholesterol.

Individuals who are very inactive receive the most benefit from an increase in exercise because exercise quickly reverses the detrimental health-related consequences of extreme inactivity, Dr. Haskell says.

In spite of a proliferation of popular books and TV commercials promoting exercise and fitness, large numbers of people remain inactive, observes Dr. Haskell. He adds, "National statistics show that 80 percent of men over 40 do not participate in any regular vigorous exercise."

Because such individuals are unable to identify with television ads that feature slim people who are models of physical fitness, such ads are a "major deterrent to getting people to exercise," Dr. Haskell suggests. These ads "lead to the perception that to get any benefit you must achieve and look like that," he says.

However, any regular activity produces substantial health-related benefits, says Dr. Haskell.

Exercise Basics and Exercise Log

He proposes that health professionals broaden exercise prescriptions to include low-intensity exercise regimens, focused on burning calories. This he believes, would bring the health benefits of regular exercise to larger numbers of people.

LIVE IT! AN EXERCISE LOG

Introduction

My walking program began in October 1984. After a few months of walking, I progressed to a walk-jog program and eventually began running. The use of a log to record my progress has not only encouraged and inspired me but has served as a record of steady progress toward my own personal fitness goals.

We have included at the top of the page a scripture for each week. You might commit these scriptures to memory. They are all promises from the Bible just for you. Let God's Word bless you as your temple becomes fit.

The Guidelines for Cardiovascular-Respiratory Training and the twelve-week charts for various aerobic exercises were used by permission Dr. Dick Couey, author of *Happiness Is Being a Physically Fit Christian*. If you will follow Dr. Couey's guidelines, you should be able to obtain the proper CVR level in a 12-week period.

Guidelines For Cardiovascular-Respiratory (CVR) Training

Probably the worst thing you can do to begin your CVR program is grab your old tennis shoes, head for the nearest track, and run at top speed. That could cause more harm than good. You must prepare yourself physically before you rush into cardiovascular exercise, or someone may have to rush you to the hospital. Please follow these guidelines and protect yourself from harm and injury.

FIRST PLACE

1. Get a medical examination, especially if you are over thirty-five years of age. The medical examination should consist of a standard and stress electrocardiogram (ECG); resting and exercise blood pressure measurements; fasting blood sugar (glucose), cholesterol, triglyceride, and high-density lipoprotein determinations; and evaluation of any orthopedic problem.
2. Warm up before exercising. Before beginning a CVR training program, subject your total body to a proper warm up. The warm up is a precaution against unnecessary injuries and muscle soreness. It stimulates the heart and lungs moderately and progressively, as well as increases the blood flow and the blood and muscle temperatures gradually. It also prepares you mentally for the approaching strenuous workout.

    The following five-minute warm-up routine is recommended. During the first two minutes, do stretching exercises for arms, legs, and back. During the third and fourth minutes, do sit-ups, push-ups, and back raisers. During the final minute, walk or jog very slowly. Strive to walk or jog flat-footed as much as possible during the warm up. This gives the tendons and ligaments in the feet and ankles a chance to stretch gradually, helping to avoid possible irritation from sudden stress.
3. Cool down after exercise. Cool down is a tapering-off period after completion of the main workout and is as important to the body as the warm up. During the CVR exercise, the large muscles of the legs provide a boost to the circulating blood and help return it to the heart and lungs where the exchange of oxygen and carbon dioxide takes place. As the muscle relaxes after exertion, blood fills the veins. It is not allowed to flow backward because of the valves in the veins. During exercise the squeezing action of the leg muscles provides about half of the pumping action, while the heart provides the other half. Walking or slow jogging, as in the cool down, allows the muscle pump to continue to work until the total volume of blood

Exercise Basics and Exercise Log

being pumped is decreased to where the heart can handle it without help from the muscles.

Always reduce your exercise pace very slowly, never abruptly. Do not stop instantly or sit down after you finish vigorous exercise or the blood will pool in your legs and you can faint from lack of blood to the brain.

4. Exercise within your tolerance. Do not push yourself to the extent of becoming overly tired. This is not only dangerous to your health, but defeats the purpose of exercise. If your body does not feel strong when you first awake, then you may be overtraining.
5. Progress slowly. In exercise, hurrying your fitness development does not work; it merely invites trouble, such as muscle and joint injuries. You do not have to be first in everything you do. Take your time in your development of fitness. Gradually work up to your exercise goals.
6. Get adequate rest and nutrition. Your body may suffer from chronic fatigue if nutrition and rest are inadequate. No matter how hard or long you train the CVR system, optimal results will not be achieved if nutrition and rest are poor.
7. Exercise regularly. Consistency and regularity are necessary for strengthening the CVR system. Spasmodic exercise can be dangerous. Your body is similar to a busy warehouse which is constantly moving goods in and out. Your exercise benefits cannot be stored; you need to add benefits daily. For every one week you cease to exercise, it takes nearly two weeks to regain the previous fitness level. Just as food intake is used up almost daily, so are the benefits of exercise unless they are replenished with more exercise.
8. Wear proper shoes. A faulty pair of exercise shoes can erase your good intentions to exercise as well as cause foot, leg, or hip injuries. Good shoes can eliminate many of the hazards associated with walking or jogging, such as blisters and stress to the feet, legs, and hips. Canvas tennis shoes are not good for walking

and jogging, because they are too heavy and usually give poor foot support to the ligaments and bones. The training type of shoe used by most long-distance runners is recommended for jogging. These have a leather or nylon upper; a good, cushioned, multilayered, spongelike sole; and a strong heel counter. Quality is the key here. Exercise participants should buy the best shoe they can afford. Anyone unsure about what shoes to purchase would be wise to consult with someone who does a lot of long-distance running.

9. Exercise cautiously in hot weather. Never exercise vigorously when a combined temperature and humidity reach 165 or above (that is, 85 degrees F. and 80 percent humidity). Exercising over this recommended rate increases susceptibility to heat stroke. Never allow your body temperature to elevate above 105 degrees F. The best method of cooling your body during exercise is through evaporation. If humidity is above 80 percent, the evaporative processes of the body do not function properly, because the humid atmosphere cannot accept any more moisture that would come from the body. The body temperature will quickly rise above the danger level. If you live in a hot and humid climate, you may have to exercise early in the morning or late at night. Wear clothes that allow your body to cool itself by evaporation. Never wear a sweat suit or rubberized suit that promotes sweating. Do not try to lose weight by sweating it off. This is not only dangerous, but you will gain the weight back when you drink fluids.

10. Dress appropriately in cold conditions. Most people overdress when they exercise in cold temperatures. Dress to feel comfortably warm during the exercise period without profuse sweating. Usually, one or two layers of light clothing, a knit cap covering the head and ears, and knit gloves are sufficient. In very cold weather, a ski mask can be worn to protect the face and warm the air as it goes into the lungs. Always run with the wind in the latter stages of your exercise. The chill factor is increased when

Exercise Basics and Exercise Log

you run into the wind. If you run against the wind after sweating has increased, the chilling effects of the wind will be magnified.

Regular systemic CVR exercise is an important key to a happy life, as it promotes physical, mental, psychological, and social fitness. It provides an outlet for emotional tensions and promotes self-confidence, wholesome social activity, and good sportsmanship. It enhances the sense of general well-being that provides the willpower to confront and master the difficult personal challenges faced each day. But remember to heed these safety precautions: start slowly, progress slowly, and do not overdo.

Walking Program

The walking program is for beginners or for individuals who have been inactive for four weeks or longer. These individuals should start with a walking program to slowly develop the leg muscles, ligaments, and tendons to prevent painful stress injuries. Hastening development by running too early only delays training because of time lost due to injuries. Furthermore, if activity is too strenuous at the start, previous ligament or joint problems could be aggravated, further delaying development.

For older people and those with a low level of CVR condition, walking initially provides enough physical stress to increase CVR fitness. If you are in poor physical condition because of prior inactivity or obesity, heed the following suggestions:

Begin walking at a normal, easy, steady pace. Swing your arms rhythmically, take in a deep breath on every fifth breath and release the air as much as possible. Acquire good jogging shoes, making sure to land on your heel first at foot strike. After several weeks, or as you become accustomed to walking, increase your speed to the point of walking a mile in fifteen minutes or less. If you cannot maintain a brisk pace, periodically slow up for several seconds, then return to your more intense pace. After you have reached an intensity level of forty-five minutes (at a pace of fifteen minutes a mile), and providing you have no joint injuries, you can begin a walk-jog-walk program.

Walking Program

Week	Walk (min.)	Frequency per week
1	15	4
2	15	5
3	18	5
4	20	5
5	23	5
6	25	5
7	28	5
8	30	5
9	33	5
10	35	5
11	40	5
12	45	5

By the end of the eighth week, you should be able to maintain a fifteen-minute mile pace.

Walk-Jog-Walk Program

The walk-jog-walk technique of training represents the simplest approach for starting an exercise program to develop CVR fitness. This program has proven successful with school children, college students, medium-age adults, and even senior adults.

Jogging is defined by most exercise physiologists as running at a pace equivalent to an eight-to-twelve-minute mile. A brisk walk is defined as walking at a pace equivalent to a twelve-to-fifteen-minute mile.

To begin your walk-jog-walk program, walk briskly for ten minutes. Then begin jogging at a pace comfortable to your level of fitness. (A comfortable pace is one in which you could carry on a short-sentence conversation as you jog without interruptions from rapid breathing.) Jog for five minutes; then cool down by walking at a slower pace for eight minutes.

Exercise Basics and Exercise Log

Walk-Jog-Walk Program

Week	Walk (min.)	Jog (min.)	Walk (min.)	Frequency per week
1	10	5	8	4
2	10	5	8	5
3	10	6	8	5
4	10	7	8	5
5	10	8	8	5
6	8	10	8	5
7	8	12	8	5
8	8	14	8	5
9	8	16	8	5
10	6	18	8	5
11	5	20	8	5
12	5	20	8	5

Check your pulse rate, making sure you reach your target heart rate of 70 percent.

Running Program

The running program is designed for individuals who want to progress further than the walk-jog-walk program or for well-conditioned individuals. The running program is designed for individuals who can run between a five- and eight-minute mile pace. So do not begin this program if you have been inactive for three weeks or longer. Progress slowly and enjoy your conditioning.

FIRST PLACE

Running Program

Week	Walk (min.)	Run (min.)	Walk (min.)	Frequency per week
1	3	20	5	5
2	3	20	5	5
3	3	22	5	5
4	3	22	5	5
5	3	25	5	5
6	3	25	5	5
7	3	28	5	5
8	3	28	5	5
9	3	32	5	5
10	3	35	5	5
11	3	40	5	5
12	3	40	5	5

Your running intensity should elevate your heart rate to the 70 percent level or higher.

Bicycling Program

To achieve a training effect with a bicycle, you must cycle slightly over twice as fast as you run to produce the same exercise heart rate. For bicycling to provide a heart rate stimulus of 70 percent of the difference between the maximum and resting rate. Also, warm up by cycling slowly for three minutes before attempting the specified time. Cool down by cycling slowly for three minutes at the conclusion of exercise.

Exercise Basics and Exercise Log

Bicycling Program

Week	Warm Up (min.)	Cycling Time (min.)	Cool Down (min.)	Frequency per week
1	3	15:00	3	5
2	3	15:00	3	5
3	3	18:00	3	5
4	3	20:00	3	5
5	3	23:00	3	5
6	3	25:00	3	5
7	3	28:00	3	5
8	3	30:00	3	5
9	3	33:00	3	5
10	3	35:00	3	5
11	3	38:00	3	5
12	3	40:00	3	5

Adjust the bicycle seat to the position in which your extended leg has a slight bend at the knee joint.

Swimming Program

Many exercise physiologists and medical authorities advocate swimming as an ideal CVR conditioner. In comparison to jogging, there is less susceptibility to injury to the leg joints. Also, the upper body muscles are worked harder for greater muscle development. Disadvantages are the accessibility of a pool and availability of an open lane that will enable you to swim unbothered.

Continuous swimming is most beneficial for improving CVR fitness. Develop your endurance to the point where you can swim the length of the pool nonstop for several minutes. You may want to use different strokes. Changing strokes systematically will strengthen all the muscles used for the different movements in the various strokes.

Check your pulse rate after a series of swims, making sure that it is at the 70 percent intensity level. Be sure to first warm up by walking back and forth across the shallow end of the pool for a minimum of three minutes. Cool down by walking in the same manner. For comparison, 100 yards of swimming equals approximately 400 yards of jogging. Therefore, jogging two miles is equivalent to about a half mile of swimming.

Swimming Program

Week	Warm Up (min.)	Swimming Time (min.)	Cool Down (min.)	Frequency per week
1	3	8:00	3	5
2	3	8:00	3	5
3	3	10:00	3	5
4	3	12:00	3	5
5	3	15:00	3	5
6	3	18:00	3	5
7	3	20:00	3	5
8	3	23:00	3	5
9	3	25:00	3	5
10	3	25:00	3	5
11	3	28:00	3	5
12	3	30:00	3	5

Wear swim goggles to protect your eyes from chemical irritants in the pool water.

Exercise Basics and Exercise Log

KNOW YOUR TRAINING HEART RATE

Aerobics: "With Oxygen" refers to exercises with one common goal: to stimulate and condition the heart, lungs, and blood vessels to their fullest capacity, thus strengthening the cardiovascular system.

Results: The heart muscle is strengthened, breathing becomes deeper, blood vessels are opened to carry more oxygen and blood to working muscles. Muscles are toned, digestion is aided, and calories are burned!

Age	Maximum Heart Rate (Beats Per Min.)	Training Heart Rate (75% Of Mhr)	Training Heart Range (70-85 Of Mhr)
20	200	150	140-170
25	195	146	137-166
30	190	142	133-162
35	185	139	130-157
40	180	135	126-153
45	175	131	123-149
50	170	127	119-145
55	165	124	116-140
60	160	120	112-136
65	155	116	109-132
70	150	112	105-128

To be in good cardiovascular health, an individual must move continuously at his or her training heart range for a minimum of 20-25 minutes 3 to 4 times a week.

Take Your Pulse: Use your first two fingers (not your thumb). Press lightly on your radial artery, close to your thumb on the inside of your wrist, or on your carotid artery, straight down from the corner of your eye, just under your chin. Count the number of beats for 10 seconds. Multiply by 6 to make sure you are within your training zone.

FIRST PLACE

During workouts, take your pulse when you start breathing hard. If you are below your zone, work a bit harder. Take your pulse every 5 to 10 minutes. If you go over your training heart rate, your exercise becomes anaerobic. You are no longer burning fat, you are burning lean body mass.

Exercise Basics and Exercise Log

But my God shall supply all your need according to his riches in glory by Christ Jesus. Philippians 4:19 (KJV)

	DATE	EXERCISE	DISTANCE	TIME	MY THOUGHTS TODAY
M					
T					
W					
T					
F					
S					
S					
	WEEK'S TOTAL				
	WEEK'S AVERAGE				
WEEK # ___	YEAR-TO-DATE				

FIRST PLACE

*Thy word is a lamp unto my feet,
and a light unto my path.* Psalm 119:105 (KJV)

	DATE	EXERCISE	DISTANCE	TIME	MY THOUGHTS TODAY
M					
T					
W					
T					
F					
S					
S					
	WEEK'S TOTAL				
	WEEK'S AVERAGE				
WEEK # ___	YEAR-TO-DATE				

Exercise Basics and Exercise Log

And whatsoever ye shall ask in my name, that will I do, that the Father may be glorified in the Son. John 14:13 (KJV)

	DATE	EXERCISE	DISTANCE	TIME	MY THOUGHTS TODAY
M					
T					
W					
T					
F					
S					
S					
	WEEK'S TOTAL				
	WEEK'S AVERAGE				
WEEK # ___	YEAR-TO-DATE				

FIRST PLACE

Not that we are sufficient of ourselves to think anything as of ourselves; but our sufficiency is of God. 2 Corinthians 3:5 (KJV)

	DATE	EXERCISE	DISTANCE	TIME	MY THOUGHTS TODAY
M					
T					
W					
T					
F					
S					
S					
	WEEK'S TOTAL				
	WEEK'S AVERAGE				
WEEK # ___	YEAR-TO-DATE				

Exercise Basics and Exercise Log

The Lord knoweth how to deliver the godly out of temptations, . . . 2 Peter 2:9a (KJV)

	DATE	EXERCISE	DISTANCE	TIME	MY THOUGHTS TODAY
M					
T					
W					
T					
F					
S					
S					
	WEEK'S TOTAL				
	WEEK'S AVERAGE				
WEEK # ___	YEAR-TO-DATE				

FIRST PLACE

Peace I leave with you, my peace I give unto you: not as the world giveth, give I unto you. Let not your heart be troubled, neither let it be afraid. John 14:27 (KJV)

	DATE	EXERCISE	DISTANCE	TIME	MY THOUGHTS TODAY
M					
T					
W					
T					
F					
S					
S					
	WEEK'S TOTAL				
	WEEK'S AVERAGE				
WEEK # ___	YEAR-TO-DATE				

Exercise Basics and Exercise Log

*I can do all things through Christ
which strengtheneth me. Philippians 4:13 (KJV)*

	DATE	EXERCISE	DISTANCE	TIME	MY THOUGHTS TODAY
M					
T					
W					
T					
F					
S					
S					
	WEEK'S TOTAL				
	WEEK'S AVERAGE				
WEEK # ___	YEAR-TO-DATE				

FIRST PLACE

*And Jesus said unto them, I am the bread of life:
he that cometh to me shall never hunger; and
he that believeth on me shall never thirst. John 6:35 (KJV)*

	DATE	EXERCISE	DISTANCE	TIME	MY THOUGHTS TODAY
M					
T					
W					
T					
F					
S					
S					
	WEEK'S TOTAL				
	WEEK'S AVERAGE				
WEEK # ___	YEAR-TO-DATE				

Exercise Basics and Exercise Log

But they that wait upon the Lord shall renew their strength; they shall mount up with wings as eagles; they shall run, and not be weary; and they shall walk, and not faint. Isaiah 40:31 (KJV)

	DATE	EXERCISE	DISTANCE	TIME	MY THOUGHTS TODAY
M					
T					
W					
T					
F					
S					
S					
	WEEK'S TOTAL				
	WEEK'S AVERAGE				
WEEK # ___	YEAR-TO-DATE				

FIRST PLACE

Beloved, I wish above all things that thou mayest prosper and be in health, even as thy soul prospereth. 3 John 2 (KJV)

	DATE	EXERCISE	DISTANCE	TIME	MY THOUGHTS TODAY
M					
T					
W					
T					
F					
S					
S					
WEEK'S TOTAL					
WEEK'S AVERAGE					
WEEK # ___ YEAR-TO-DATE					

Exercise Basics and Exercise Log

But without faith it is impossible to please him; for he that cometh to God must believe that he is, and that he is a rewarder of them that diligently seek him. Hebrews 11:6 (KJV)

	DATE	EXERCISE	DISTANCE	TIME	MY THOUGHTS TODAY
M					
T					
W					
T					
F					
S					
S					
	WEEK'S TOTAL				
	WEEK'S AVERAGE				
WEEK # ___	YEAR-TO-DATE				

FIRST PLACE

*Therefore if any man be in Christ,
he is a new creature: old things are passed away;
behold, all things are become new. 2 Corinthians 5:17 (KJV)*

	DATE	EXERCISE	DISTANCE	TIME	MY THOUGHTS TODAY
M					
T					
W					
T					
F					
S					
S					
WEEK'S TOTAL					
WEEK'S AVERAGE					
WEEK # ___ YEAR-TO-DATE					

APPENDIX H

Sample Bible Study

WEEK 1: GIVING CHRIST FIRST PLACE

Memory verse
"But seek first his kingdom and his righteousness, and all these things will be given to you as well." Matthew 6:33

In Matthew 22:37, we discover the place God wants to hold in our lives: "Love the Lord your God with all your heart and with all your soul and with all your mind."

What a challenge! It's not enough to love God halfheartedly. Offering Him part of our lives isn't enough. He wants all, our complete commitment. Christ wants "first place" so every area of our lives is under His control.

This week in your study, you'll have the opportunity to search your heart and examine your life. Are there areas of your life you have failed to surrender to Christ? If Christ is not first place in your thoughts, plans, and actions, what is?

Day 1: Time for what you seek first

Matthew 6:33 contains the pattern for Christian living in a nutshell: "Seek first the kingdom of God." We live busy lives. We cannot do everything. Often, the only thing we can decide is what we will do first. What we choose first, over time, becomes first place in our lives.

Think back over the last month of your life. What do your calendar and your checkbook suggest has been first place in your life in that period of time?

_____
_____
_____

God knows that things other than spiritual priorities tend to become the focus of our lives. Our checkbooks and calendars remind us of this fact.

In Matthew 6:25, Jesus mentions some of the things that divert our attention from His priorities for our lives. List them.

_____
_____
_____

Day 7: Evidence that Christ is first place

As Christians, we should desire to give Christ first place in every area of our lives. Saying Christ is first and living with Christ in first place are different matters. When Christ comes first, life changes. We make decisions based on new commitments. We schedule time based on new priorities.

The following verses describe some of the priorities and commitments that indicate we have given Christ first place. Look up each verse and match the verse with the key phrase to the left:[1]

Characteristic in our lives	Scripture
___ 1. a desire and willingness to obey God	A. Proverbs 3:9–10
___ 2. offering yourself to God as a living sacrifice	B. 1 Thessalonians 5:17
___ 3. giving to God from our material possessions	C. Romans 13:8
___ 4. loving others on an ongoing basis	D. Romans 12:1
___ 5. an ongoing lifestyle of prayer	E. 1 Samuel 15:22

Sample Bible Study

Based on these verses, how would you evaluate the degree to which Christ is first place in your life right now? Check the box beside each characteristic that best expresses the degree to which that characteristic is developed in your life:

This characteristic in my life is...	strong	average	weak
I desire to know and obey God.	❏	❏	❏
I offer myself to God as a living sacrifice.	❏	❏	❏
I give to God from my material possessions.	❏	❏	❏
I love others on an ongoing basis.	❏	❏	❏
I sustain a lifestyle of prayer.	❏	❏	❏

In which area do you need to make the greatest changes? Are you ready to make those changes? Tell God about your desire to give Him first place in your life.

Your week in review

Of the biblical truths you studied, which has been most helpful?

_____
_____

Of the biblical truths you learned, which has been the most convicting?

_____
_____

Of the changes you need to make, which will you make first?

_____
_____
_____

[1] Answers 1-E, 2-D, 3-A, 4-C, 5-B

APPENDIX I

Additional First Place Resources

If you would like a catalog of First Place accessories for ordering, please call 1-800-727-5223.

Achieve a healthy lifestyle with Christ in first place

With *First Place: A Christ-Centered Health Program*, you'll discover that weight control is just the beginning. *First Place* helps you manage all areas of your life by incorporating a balanced, consistent approach to life through healthy eating, exercise, Bible study, prayer, and weekly accountability meetings. Through *First Place*, you can gain energy, enthusiasm, and confidence—enabling you to be the person God wants you to be.

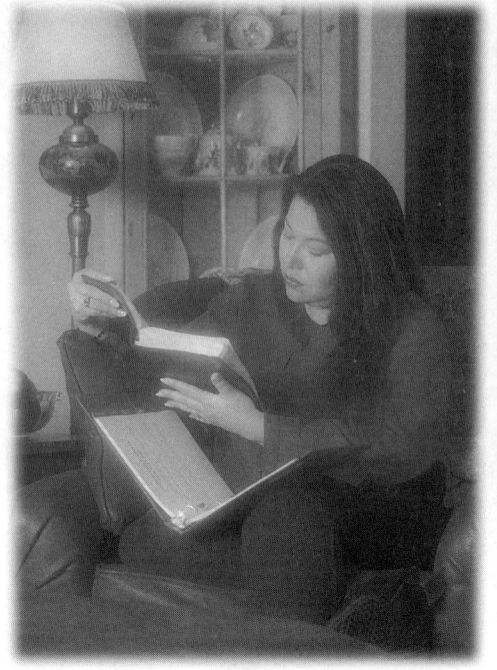

"I can do all things through Christ who strengthens me."
—*Philippians 4:13, NIV*

Each member needs:

First Place: A Christ-Centered Health Program Member's Notebook—Core materials which include handouts and health information.
0767326091 ....$44.95*

FIRST PLACE BIBLE STUDY PACK: *Giving Christ First Place*—10-week Bible study, plus a prayer journal.
0805499954 ....$14.95*

Each leader needs:

First Place Leader's Guide Includes discussion questions for the Bible studies, plus a copy of *Choosing to Change: The First Place Challenge*.
0767326105 ....$29.95*

Orientation/Food Exchange Video—Use at first meeting to explain program.
0767326121 ....$29.95*

New!
First Place for Youth—Includes leader guide, meal planner, and youth edition Bible studies.

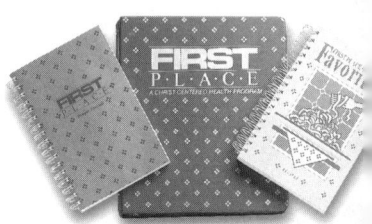

To order these small-group study resources, Write, call, or fax:
Customer Service Center; MSN 11
127 Ninth Avenue, North; Nashville
TN 37234-0113; **1-800-458-2772**

*Plus Shipping — $4.00 minimum.

ENDNOTES

Chapter One

1. John Graham, quoting Meginnis and Foege, "Actual Causes of Death in the United States," *Journal of American Medical Association*, 1993.
2. Jim Ritter, Health Science Reporter, *Chicago Sun Times*, September 18, 1997.

Chapter Three

1. Zig Ziglar, *See You at the Top*, (New York: Pelican Publishing Company, 1975), n. p.
2. Oswald Chambers, *My Utmost for His Highest: An Updated Edition in Today's Language*, edited by James Reimann, (Grand Rapids, Michigan: Discovery House Publishers, 1992). May 20.

Chapter Four

1. Patsy Clairmont, from a presentation at Highland Lakes Baptist Encampment, Austin, Texas, October, 1984.

Chapter Five

1. Ziglar, p. 288.
2. Tim Hansel, *Holy Sweat*, (Dallas: Word Publishing, 1987), p. 117.

3. Ibid, p. 157.

Chapter Six

1. William Heston, "Putting the Past in Perspective," First Place Conference, Woodmont, Georgia, 24 October, 1997.
2. *Leaves of God, An Anthology of Prayers, Memorable Phrases, Inspirational Verse and Prose*, edited by Clye Francis Lytle, (Fort Worth, Texas: Brownlow Publishing Company, Inc. 1938), p. 108.

Chapter Eight

1. Bill Hybels, *Honest to God*, (Grand Rapids, Michigan: Zondervan Publishing, 1990), pp. 169-171.
2. Ibid.